DEVELOPING AND MANAGING
HIGH QUALITY SERVICES FOR PEOPLE WITH
LEARNING DISABILITIES

To all Manchester's learning-disabled people, their families and the staff who support them.

Developing and Managing High Quality Services for People with Learning Disabilities

Edited by
Mark Burton
and
Mike Kellaway

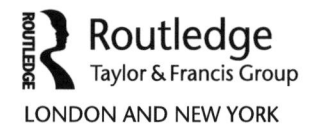
Routledge
Taylor & Francis Group

LONDON AND NEW YORK

First published 1998 by Ashgate Publishing

Reissued 2018 by Routledge
2 Park Square, Milton Park, Abingdon, Oxon, OX14 4RN
711 Third Avenue, New York, NY 10017, USA

Routledge is an imprint of the Taylor & Francis Group, an informa business

Publisher's Note
The publisher has gone to great lengths to ensure the quality of this reprint but points out that some imperfections in the original copies may be apparent.

Disclaimer
The publisher has made every effort to trace copyright holders and welcomes correspondence from those they have been unable to contact.

A Library of Congress record exists under LC control number: 97049091

ISBN 13: 978-1-138-31285-2 (hbk)
ISBN 13: 978-0-429-45798-2 (ebk)

Contents

List of figures

List of tables

List of contributors

The contributors are all staff of the Joint Learning Disability Service in Manchester, employed either by The Mancunian Community Health NHS Trust, or by the City of Manchester Social Services Department.

Editors

Mark Burton   Head of Development and Clinical Services
Mike Kellaway Head of Joint Learning Disability Service

Other contributors

Christine Adcock	Clinical Psychologist
Allen Briscoe	Network Manager
Ian Crabtree	Practice Advisor, Occupational Therapy
Dave Crier	Assistant Network Manager
Bernie Gibbins	Community Learning Disability Team Manager
Karen Goodman	Quality Development Officer
Nigel Hoar	Assistant Network Manager
Pauline John	Area Manager
Jane Jolliffe	Practice Advisor, Speech and Language Therapy
Phil Jones	Clinical Manager
Sylvia Jones	Speech and Language Therapist
Lynsay Juffs	Speech and Language Therapist
Jean Lally	Clinical Psychologist
Iain Larkin	Network Manager

Cathi McKessy	Occupational Therapist
Maxine Martin	Community Learning Disability Team Manager
Jude Moss	Clinical Psychologist
Mike Petrou	Network Manager
Andrew Pope	Project Leader: Complex Needs Day Service
Linda Prinsloo	Occupational Therapist
Dave Ruane	Residential Manager
Rachel Samuels	Speech and Language Therapist
Helen Sanderson	Quality Development Officer
Moira Speechley	Occupational Therapist
Debbie Windley	Occupational Therapist

List of abbreviations

ANM	assistant network manager
CLDT	community learning disability team
ELP	Essential Lifestyle Planning
GAS	Goal Attainment Scaling
IPP	Individual Programme Plan
LETS	Local Exchange Trading Scheme
PAM	profession ancillary to medicine
QAG	quality action group
RSW	residential social worker
SI	sensory integration
TAG	training action group

Foreword

The challenges facing services for people with learning disabilities have probably never been greater for those managing and providing them as well as for those using them. The climate is one of financial retrenchment with little hope of relief. There is the prospect of further structural change as trust mergers and service reconfigurations gather pace. The shifting, though often unfocused, boundary between primary and community care, and between this and secondary care, creates confusion and uncertainty for everyone and can compound low morale among staff who already feel insecure and vulnerable.

Under the weight of such pressures, it would be all too easy, if understandable, to become negative about the future and to feel disempowered and overwhelmed by the sense that it is all too difficult and rather pointless. For those in that position, this book should serve as something of a tonic, offering hope in the midst of despair and despondency.

The authors do not evade the difficult problems and pressures they confronted in setting up the Joint Learning Disability Service in Manchester but they are able somehow to convey an abiding optimism and deep commitment to their work which not only shines through the book but allows them, and their colleagues, to find solutions to the problems facing them and to make a difference.

Evidence of this commitment and obvious enthusiasm is the appearance of this book which is unusual in that it is written by those whose job it is to manage and provide the Joint Learning Disability Service. In the academic literature much is made of the need for practitioners to stand back and reflect on their work and to communicate something of the flavour of life on the front line at a time of change. The fact that few practitioners manage to find the time or have the energy or inclination to achieve this makes this book particularly welcome and can only strengthen its appeal.

I first discovered the Joint Learning Disability Service in 1995 when I was invited to join the panel of judges for the *Health Service Journal* Management Awards. The Service had been shortlisted in the community and primary care category and it was the entry I chose to visit. I did not regret it. More importantly, it subsequently gave me great pleasure to see the Service win the award in its category against tough competition.

My brief visit could not do justice to the complexities and subtleties of the Service. But I was struck by the overall positive atmosphere, commitment, sense of purpose and sheer energy of the staff I met. There was clearly goodwill on all sides in negotiating problems, getting round red tape and bureaucracy, and putting users' preferences uppermost. What was particularly impressive about the Service was its jointness. In my notes on the visit I wrote: 'as far as a joint service was concerned there was no issue about the health/social care divide – it simply did not exist'. The central focus was on the user and their needs with the specialist expertise and staff skills coalescing, as appropriate, to meet them.

It had not always been like that, however, with a 'Berlin Wall' in evidence between health and social services. While the wall had been dismantled, it was acknowledged that tensions between the different perspectives persisted. But these were regarded as a positive feature contributing to the whole being greater than the sum of the parts. The blending of skills in place of tribalistic rituals and warring factions was an impressive feature of the initiative. Much is to be heard these days about joint commissioning, rather less about joint provision despite its obvious importance in terms of realising truly seamfree care.

So this book is most welcome as it provides a detailed and honest account of the Joint Learning Disability Service's genesis and evolution. It is full of important insights and lessons for managers, practitioners and users as well as policy-makers. Two stand out for me. First, the editors, while acknowledging the limitations of large public organisations, add:

> ... but we also know that they do not have to function in an unimaginative bureaucratic way. We have yet to be convinced of the advantage of their replacement with a patchwork of small providers, operating in an imitation of a market.

Second, the importance of leadership and good management is stressed so that responsibility is taken 'for ensuring that good things happen and bad practice is identified and stopped'. Most crucial of all, 'authority to create real change is often there for the taking'. Regrettably, such leadership and management remain the exception rather than the rule.

The authors are not complacent but they have a good story to tell, which they do with confidence and a conviction that their experiences can be of value to others. Lesson-learning is a vital part of staff and organisational development. This book repays careful study in that it may help spawn similar services elsewhere. There is nothing mystical about the reasons for success. Nor need they be confined to services for people with learning disabilities.

David J. Hunter
Professor of Health Policy and Management
Nuffield Institute for Health
University of Leeds

Note to readers

Authors can be contacted at the following address, which is also the address for ordering publications of the Joint Service cited in the text.

Joint Learning Disability Service
Chapman Place
Chapman St
Gorton
Manchester
M18 8UA
Tel: 0161 223 9901
Fax: 0161 223 7792

Introduction

This book is for people involved in services for people with learning disabilities. It has been written by managers and staff in Manchester's Joint Learning Disability Service, and its primary readership is people like ourselves – managers and staff in learning disability services. We also hope that the book will be of interest and relevance for a variety of other people These include:

- *Parents and other relatives of learning-disabled people,* who often feel kept in the dark regarding the world of human services and who might wish to use some of the examples in this book when trying to obtain appropriate provision for their relatives.
- *People involved in independent advocacy for people with learning disabilities,* who need to have some examples of what is possible, and to have some counterarguments to use when they are told that some things are 'not possible'.
- *Those in commissioning roles,* who are often underresourced for their strategic tasks and who are not always specialists in the learning disability field. This book might help define some desirable goals for principled commissioning and purchasing on behalf of learning-disabled people.
- *Those involved in the education and training of people who do, or who will, work in these services.*
- *Researchers* who need an overview of service provision issues within which to contextualise their work.
- *Those with roles in inspection, accreditation or consultancy with services.* The availability of some models of good practice, and of some developmental strategies that have been used effectively, should help in

xxiv *Developing and Managing Services for People with Learning Disabilities*

both establishing standards and in helping other organisations improve their performance.

- *Those involved in formulating policy.* The current division of labour between the various organisations in the social welfare field is but one possible permutation. The splits between purchaser and provider, statutory and voluntary, health and social care, for example, are all contestable. This book will help in the development of policy and organisational design as the most recent changes in the human services are appraised.
- *People with primary interests in other areas of health and welfare provision,* for whom the broad lessons of this book will also be relevant.

The chapters generally follow a similar format. First, the topic is introduced and put into context. Then key issues are identified in order to give a concept to the topic. This is followed by practical guidance which is intended to orientate the reader towards some useful activities. Finally, experience and examples from our service in Manchester are described, to make concrete the analysis and advice in earlier sections, and also to demonstrate what is possible.

In Manchester we made an interesting and unusual attempt to produce broad-scale principled service change and development across the main provider agencies. This is the Joint Learning Disability Service, which as Chapter 1 explains, is an alliance, established in 1994, between the City of Manchester Social Services Department and the Mancunian Community Health NHS Trust (Burton and Kellaway, 1995). From a very patchy base we have come a long way in increasing the effectiveness and quality of our services. We are by no means complacent, but we think we have discovered some promising 'roads to quality' in the way that we have configured, developed, managed and provided our services. What may be learned from our experience has applicability beyond learning disability services as such, and our joint provision experiment has relevance to policy for both health and social services

The editors and writers have tried to strike a balance between analysis, theory and conceptualisation, on the one hand, and the Manchester story on the other. This has not always been easy: many of the contributors initially found it difficult to identify the underlying issues, rather than write about their experience. The editors have helped with this, sometimes drafting more conceptual sections, sometimes supplying what became known as 'essay plans' for the writers to follow. We hope that this has resulted in a book which offers some helpful conceptual frameworks and guidance to those trying to promote high-quality provision, while continually grounding both ideas and recommendations in experience that has been hard-won in circumstances that can be as constraining as those anywhere else in the country.

The material covered is inevitably selective: we have written about the areas we are familiar with, and these cover many of the key issues in improving opportunities for people who are learning-disabled. Some obvious areas are not covered: adult placement and life-sharing models, supported employment, care management, psychiatric provision are examples.

The assumptions we make in compiling this book are presented below in the form of key themes that will be met throughout the book in various guises:

1 *The importance of the values of public service and responsible citizenship.* People with learning disability are relatively vulnerable. They also have great potential to contribute to society and to live fulfilling lives. For this to happen they need a sound basis of accountable and publicly funded services. The book should illustrate a combination of an entrepreneurial spirit with an emphasis on fairness, cooperation and finding ways to safeguard people's interests without constraining their lives. We work in large public organisations and know their limitations, but we also know that they do not have to function in an unimaginative bureaucratic way. We have yet to be convinced of the advantage of their replacement with a patchwork of small providers, operating in an imitation of a market. Our experience suggests that the contribution of small independent providers is most effective when they work in partnership with provider organisations that can assist them with training, practice development, and logistic support (see Towell, 1996 and Cambridge and Brown, 1997 for a related viewpoint).

2 *The indivisibility of needs.* Formal and *de facto* lead responsibility in services for people with learning disabilities has shifted back and forth between health and social services authorities over the years. For the last 15 years there has been considerable collaboration in joint planning and management, and in the transfer of clients and resources between organisations. With the shift to community provision, much professional expertise has been 'left behind' in the NHS, sometimes marooned in single-agency teams which can become isolated from the rest of service provision.

One much canvassed resolution to the problems of the split service has been the joint commissioning of services. However, in Manchester an alternative approach to collaboration has been developed – joint provision. This is thought to address one of the key issues directly – that of the interrelatedness of the work of supporting people with significant learning disabilities effectively in the community. In day-to-day work we do not ask if something is a health or social issue, but recognise the interplay between the two. Health depends on social supports, which in turn depend on health: '*You can't see the join*' – or at least you shouldn't be able to. We are therefore not very interested in debates between so called 'medical models' and 'social models' of disability, but instead seek to put the specialised skills of professionals into a context where they make a relevant contribution to people's everyday well-being and life experience, without dominating the nature of that experience. Our chief tools in doing this are clarity about what we are all trying to achieve, and effective management of the service (which includes the deployment of resources, the guidance and equipping of staff, and the operation of effective safeguards to protect the interests of those who rely on service supports).

3 *The importance of community.* Reciprocity, belonging and being important to someone are perhaps the things that help us to be fully human. It is difficult to see how these can exist if people are isolated and segregated. We have lived and worked through a major change in the north-west – the bringing home of thousands of people with learning disabilities to various kinds of supported ordinary existence in the community. That process has taught us the importance of having a principled stance on matters such as group size, and backing that stance with financial incentives to providers. Our work, and the orientation of this book, emphasises the centrality of assisting people to lead real lives in real communities. We don't think that this can be compromised, even if there have to be compromises on some aspects of the realisation: some people might have to live in groups of four, but that doesn't mean they shouldn't live in a house in a street, be known by the neighbours or the person in the corner shop, have people call, go to concerts, take a trip on a canal boat or visit local restaurants.

4 *The importance of leadership and good management.* Good things don't just happen by themselves. Those in leadership positions (and that doesn't just mean managers) have to take responsibility for ensuring that good things happen and that bad practice is identified and stopped. Our experience suggests that authority to create real change is often there for the taking and, in the absence of such initiative, services and the people who rely on them will languish. Perhaps the most important thing is to provide encouragement for staff initiative: most people want to do a good job, and most people have good ideas. Real progress depends on unlocking that source of energy and creativity within a shared set of values and parameters. This book is full of examples of initiatives which had their origin in a staff member's good idea. It may be objected that we are stating the obvious but, if this is so, then why is this type of

leadership and management not the norm? This book is intended to offer some guidelines for service providers who want to do better.

The creation of this book has been one of those bright ideas that generate a great deal of extra work. Much of this work has been carried out in people's own time, and the editors are grateful to all the contributors. We are also grateful to our families for their support and to the senior officers of both organisations for their continual support for the Joint Service and our attempt to make it something of which Manchester can be proud.

Mark Burton
Mike Kellaway

References

Burton, M. and Kellaway, M (1995), 'Specialisation without separation: combining health and social services provision for people with learning disabilities', *Health and Social Care in the Community*, 3 (4), 263–67.

Cambridge, P. and Brown, H. (1997), 'Making the market work for people with learning disabilities: an argument for principled contracting', *Critical Social Policy*, 17 (2), 27–52.

Towell, D. (1996), 'Revaluing the NHS: empowering ourselves to shape a health care system fit for the 21st century', *Policy and Politics* 24, 287–97.

Part I

Organisational Issues

Introduction

The two chapters in this Part, both by Mark Burton and Mike Kellaway, concern the structures of the service.

Chapter 1, 'Joint Working' addresses the split in the UK between social care and health care. As might be expected, given its origin in a joint provider organisation, a key theme of this book is the indivisibility of health and social needs and issues. Although the organisational split between health and social care is by no means inevitable, in the UK the division between central and local government responsibilities tends to exacerbate it. Given this separation, joint working arrangements between health and welfare organisations become necessary if people with learning disabilities and their families are to receive coherent services. Chapter 1 reviews the issues involved in enhancing joint working and illustrates these with the development of the joint provision model in Manchester and its implementation in the Joint Service.

Chapter 2, 'Designing the Organisation', deals with the internal structure of the organisation. As Pettigrew (1986) pointed out before the last upheaval in health and social provision, changing organisational structures alone will not deliver significant benefits, but in conjunction with other 'management levers' – strategy, process, systems, beliefs and behaviour, and capability – fundamental change (for the better) can take place.

Reference

Pettigrew, A. (1986), 'Managing strategic change' in G. Parston (ed.), *Managers as Strategists: Health Services Managers Reflecting on Practice*, London: King's Fund.

1 Joint working

Mark Burton and Mike Kellaway

People with learning disabilities have many different needs. Some of these are commonplace and some are special.

> Derek is a young man in his late twenties. He is described as having a profound learning disability, but he walks and we believe that his vision and hearing are unimpaired. He lives in an ordinary house in the community and is supported by staff 24 hours a day. Staff believe that he enjoys swimming and walking. Left to his own devices Derek will do little, except acquire food and drink. He will occasionally get up and change his position. He can do little for himself, although he has learned spoon feeding, door opening and masturbation in the last 15 years. He exhibits a great deal of self-stimulatory behaviour, and this shades into head-banging, particularly when there is little to stimulate him in his immediate environment.

From the time we have spent with Derek, we have good reason to think that his needs include the following:

Ordinary needs
- nutritious food
- a comfortable house
- people that know, understand and care about him
- being in ordinary places in the community
- a guaranteed income.
- alternative activities to self-stimulation.

Special needs
- help to overcome his head-banging
- protection from dangers he does not understand
- effective teaching of new skills

Meeting needs is not the exclusive preserve of one single organisation, and our experience teaches us that people are best supported where staff with different skills, experiences, knowledge and backgrounds work closely together. In Derek's case this means deploying the 'ordinary' skills of making a comfortable, welcoming home and sustaining his relationships, in concert with the more specialist skills of analysing his repetitive behaviour and self-injury, and creating effective and sustainable interventions to reduce them. The task, then, is one of enabling the different employing organisations to work together effectively so that people with learning disabilities and their allies experience 'seamless' provision – that is, provision without artificial barriers, boundary disputes or rivalries.

However, while the idea of enabling the different organisations to work together sounds simple, it is rarely straightforward in practice. In this chapter we explore the development of joint working, consider key issues in its realisation and provide guidance on how to make it happen, with illustrations from our own experience in Manchester.

The long and slow development of joint working in the UK

In 1948 the National Health Service (NHS) was established, and provision for people with learning disabilities was reorganised. One consequence was that the 'colonies' and similar institutions which had been run by local authorities were taken into the new NHS, and, overnight, some staff were redesignated as nurses. This was followed by a period during which intellectual disability was 'medicalised', with 'mental handicap nursing' only gradually working its way into a more social and developmental model.

Meanwhile the care of those people who were not in institutions became the responsibility of the mental health departments of the local authorities. They employed mental welfare officers, and ran services such as adult and junior training centres and, eventually, hostels.

This division of labour changed slowly in the first two decades after 1948. In 1959 the new Mental Health Act heralded a policy shift towards caring for people in the community. In 1971 the 'Seebohm' reorganisation led to the establishment of local-authority social services departments, which combined a variety of functions including child protection, mental welfare and the social care of older people. In 1974 the NHS was reorganised with the establishment of regional and area health authorities, which hesitantly began to change focus from hospital provision to the meeting of health care needs on a population basis. There was some realignment of responsibilities between the NHS and local government with these two reorganisations, and the transfer of staff in both directions. Unfortunately, one consequence of 'Seebohm' was a switch in most authorities to generic social work. The skills, experience and knowledge of mental welfare officers was often lost within these new generic teams.

Other changes were taking place at the same time. Many were underpinned by a 'philosophical shift' in the way in which people with intellectual disabilities were perceived: new psychological and educational research increased expectations, the 'community option' began to become a reality in several different countries, and positive ideologies such as 'least restrictive alternative', personalisation and 'normalisation' became influential, partly in the wake of the 1960s civil rights movements. Notable developments in the UK were:

- **1971**: Government White Paper, *Better Services for the Mentally Handicapped*. Emphasised the goal of community-based provision (but in a limited way).
- **1971**: Education Act gave all children the right to education. Junior training centres were redesignated as special schools.
- **1974**: The Joint Finance scheme was established. This was a ring-fenced budget allocated to health authorities but spent jointly with local authorities. Joint planning structures were set up to make decisions.
- **1975**: A National Development Group and a National Development Team were set up following several hospital abuse scandals. The National Development Group published a report, *Teams for Mentally Handicapped People*, which recommended an interagency and interdisciplinary community learning disability team model.
- **1979**: The Jay Committee report on the future of nursing care for people with learning disabilities, influenced by the early staffed housing models, emphasised homemaking skills and proposed a merger between the registered nurse, mental handicap (RNMH) training and the Certificate of Social Services qualification. Although resisted by the nursing profession, it became influential for its model of care.

In the 1980s joint working developed slowly and to different extents between authorities. Professionals in NHS community services and in social services departments often established good working relationships despite their employing organisations. Before the mid-1980s very few NHS community-based professionals specialised in learning disability. The 1983 Care in the Community circular extended the Joint Finance scheme and also enabled health authorities to transfer funds to local authorities and the voluntary sector. This became the basis for the resettlement dowries (cash-linked with people discharged from hospitals) and gave health and social services authorities a considerable incentive to agree a vision and jointly plan to resettle people. Again, the development was uneven across the country: regions which required agreed plans between local authorities and district health authorities achieved greater commitment to, and experience of, interagency working.

Just as the joint approach seemed to be maturing at the end of the 1980s, health and social services were thrown into a period of uncertainty and upheaval with the National Health and Community Care Act 1990 which led to purchaser–provider splits, increased outsourcing in the independent sector and a loss of continuity in many areas as staff and managers changed jobs. In many areas this weakened joint working.

Key issues

Promoting joint working involves considering a number of issues, concerning what is to be attempted and what local factors will help and hinder the effort. These issues can broadly be broken down into the following:

- the degree of joint working intended
- role clarity, division of labour, overlaps and gaps
- leadership, responsibility and management
- markets and the purchaser–provider split
- the political dimension.

How joint?

What degree of joint working is to be attempted? As is shown in Table 1.1, the degree of joint working can be rated from low to high on two dimensions – staff working practices, and organisational collaboration. Table 1.1 seems to demonstrate a developmental progression from low 'jointness' to total integration, and this may be a useful perspective. However, it is sometimes possible to jump stages, if the will is there.

Role clarity, division of labour, overlaps and gaps

This issue concerns the focus of each organisation's effort. In some places health and social services have very different functions and responsibilities, while in others there can be overlap. For example, in Manchester, a decision

Table 1.1 Degrees of joint working

Rating	Staff working together	Organisations working together
Nil	Staff work entirely separately, in ignorance of each others' roles.	No liaison, duplication of functions. Ignorance of other organisation.
Low	Staff refer to one another and meet at reviews and case conferences.	Liaison at the margins (for example, through mandatory forums).
Mid	Staff involved in joint ventures such as joint training. Attempts to use common systems of case coordination, registers and so on. Increasing understanding of each others' roles.	Shared strategy but separate management: likely to be some collaborative joint problem-solving leading to flexibility of resources (for example, loan/ secondment of staff).
High	Co-location of staff, but still mostly under separate management. Staff increasingly working together as one team. Increasing respect for each other's skills.	Some experiments in full collaboration – for example, some management and coordination across organisational boundaries
Total	Staff managed together as one team.	Organisations have joint management agreement, with single manager/management team.

taken early in the 1980s led to the NHS concentrating on the provision of a variety of professionals through community teams, while social services emphasised 'hard provision' such as day services, 24-hour care, and unqualified staff providing practical support to families (as well as employing specialist social workers). As a result, the services complemented one another, and it soon became obvious that joint effectiveness would be improved by integration.

In some other nearby districts, the NHS had provided large-scale housing-based residential services and had only a minor investment in professional staff other than nurses. Meanwhile social services provided traditional hostels, newer dispersed residential services, day services and (largely generic) social workers. This resulted in a duplication of residential function and gaps in the professional and non-building-based practical care elements, making the integration of services perhaps less easy to arrange, even though it was no less desirable than in Manchester.

Leadership, responsibility and management

What can be achieved in the short term will partly depend on the leaders in both organisations. Here is a set of questions that can be asked:

- Do the leaders know each other? Do they understand one another's perspectives, concerns and agendas? How long have they worked together? Have they solved problems and made things happen together?
- Do they have the backing of their organisations – senior managers, authority or board members and their staff?
- How well do they know the service, its users and their allies?
- Do they have a vision of what it is that they are trying to achieve? (This need not (should not) be fully worked out, but should indicate the direction in which these services are to go.)
- Do they share responsibility, or do they tend to shunt responsibility on to one another?

Markets and the purchaser–provider split

The movement of health and welfare organisations into the current quasi-market mode has led to a proliferation of stakeholders – both purchasers and providers – and, with increased outsourcing to the independent sector, a rise in the number of service providers. The accountability of providers is now more complex, with answerability to both line management and purchaser interests. The implementation of purchaser–provider splits differs between health and social care: health purchasers (with the exception of GPs) have a broad-scale approach related to population need; social care purchasers typically have some responsibilities for coordination of care to individuals. Moreover, social service authorities differ from one another in how and where in the organisation they have implemented the purchaser–provider split.

The purchaser–provider splits do not make the goal of joint working and seamless supports any easier. Anyone working towards increased joint working must consider which purchaser and provider functions need to be integrated and which do not. In Manchester we have adopted a joint provision model, and joint commissioning is likely to follow. However, our (provider) care managers carry out some delegated (and monitored) purchasing functions for the local authority purchaser. Other areas have emphasised joint commissioning from the start and have only recently begun to consider how to integrate provision.

The key is to keep asking the 'So what?' question:

What will this mean for people who rely on the service?

The political dimension

To make effective progress in joint working the organisation's top leadership and other key stakeholders must have committed ownership of the task. Without this, any arrangements made risk being makeshift, interim, and potentially vulnerable. Positive responses to the following questions will reveal whether the commitment is in place.

- Do senior managers and authority and board members have a shared vision of what they want to achieve? Does this vision include people with intellectual disabilities?
- Are there strong cross-organisational links and relationships at this level?
- Is there the political will for change?
- Are staff and their representatives involved, informed and open to development and change in the interorganisational relationship, given that this might mean changes in workplaces, working practices, management arrangements, workplace culture and so on?
- Is the climate of relationships between the organisations marked by trust and respect or suspicion and dismissiveness?

Practical guidance

Structure

Organisational structure is covered in Chapter 2. However, at this point it is worth mentioning the issue of management accountability outside of the employing authority, which is inevitable in a joint service or in similar interorganisational management arrangements. This can be difficult for staff to come to terms with and, unless the lines are clear, there is the possibility of confusion and divisiveness. The key lies in building mutual trust rather than in direction and control: staff in community services have considerable minute-to-minute discretion and autonomy (the manager is not always there) so management must build and rely on consent rather than on coercion as its main mode.

Audit: mapping the provision

The incentive for services to move towards a joint model of provision usually derives from a review of the overlapping areas of each agency's work.

Services need to define and agree the population to be served. In some areas of work this will be quite straightforward: people with diabetes, for example, either have the condition or not. In others this will be more problematic. In learning disability services much energy is still spent in defining who exactly qualifies. Will it be those people who have been identified by the Education Service by attendance at schools for children with severe learning difficulties? (This is a less reliable definition now that learning-disabled children are increasingly accommodated in mainstream schools.) Will the cut-off be the first percentile of ability, or two standard deviations from the mean in the population? Or will it be one of the many other definitions, none of which quite fits the bill? It is critical that agreement is reached.

In many areas the agency wanting to move towards a joint model of working will have coterminous boundaries. Unfortunately this won't always be the case. Establishing joint working arrangements for part, but not all, of an agency's geographical area of responsibility can be fraught with difficulties. Agencies need to confront this problem and develop ways of providing services in the area not covered. This has been done for learning disability services in Tameside where the Tameside local authority boundaries are not coterminous with the Tameside and Glossop Community Trust.

Part of the mapping exercise is to plot which agency manages which part of the service. The evolutionary pattern of public services have evolved over the century and this exercise will often demonstrate that there is no reasoned basis for who does what! Local authorities, particularly in the 1970s, took on many tasks. Social services departments, more than many other local authority departments, expanded beyond their obvious remit – for example, managing homeless family accommodation which is surely a housing department function! In learning disability services, responsibility for which has swung back and forth between the local authority and health authority, the mapping exercise will often reveal much overlap. For instance, the local authority might run a day centre which transports users by bus past a day centre run by the local community health trust, even though there is no discernible difference between the users of each service.

The mapping exercise can lead to a reorganisation of responsibilities which could reflect the different skills available to each agency or the range or location of their services.

Incentives

The push towards joint working arrangements often needs help to overcome the protectionism of each agency. A major incentive to produce this new model will be finance. Agencies that operate in similar areas of work will see that there are savings to be made in management, administration and other non-pay costs. The need for learning disability services in the north-west region to reach agreement on the resettlement of people from long-stay institutions brought many health and local authorities together for the first time. Chief officers and accountants developed an understanding of the pressures on their counterparts as they struggled to resolve the issues of dowries or individual packages of care. For larger authorities the money involved was significant for all: it paved the way for collaborative problem-solving in this and other areas.

The vogue in community care is joint commissioning. Increasingly, purchasers of services are requiring services providers to work together to produce more effective outcomes for users and patients. Joint provision may be driven by commissioners or be seen by agencies as a way of securing or maintaining existing contracts.

Working from both ends: staff, users, unions, managers and members

It is unlikely that users or staff will demand joint working arrangements. More often managers of services recognise the possibilities and begin discussions or are required to do so in response to their committee or board members.

It is critical that all the stakeholders are involved – ideally, when the agenda is initially set. Local authority councillors, the Social Services Committee and the board members from the health trusts will have concerns about loss of control and accountability. Staff may view change as leading to a change of role or reduced autonomy. Unions may see joint working as a way of introducing staff cuts or downgrading of jobs. Service users and their families, who rely on the limited support systems, may fear that change will mean that each agency will reduce its services. Managers may become anxious about loss of status or job.

Consultation at an early stage may initially raise concerns but will provide a forum to develop a model which reassures those stakeholders that, although something may be given up, something richer will be gained.

It is important to achieve some early success, particularly if this is very visible. A joint training programme or shared project will demonstrate the advantages of using the skills, experience and resources of both agencies to produce a better outcome than either could do individually.

A difficult lesson to learn is that it is not possible to work jointly and be in control all the time.

Shared vision

Unless the partners in a joint working arrangement share a vision of the service to be provided, it is unlikely to be successful. It is often through the struggle – the debate or argument about what a quality service would look like – that the seed of joint working germinates.

In learning disability services it has been generally accepted that an ordinary life model is the preferred model of care. It is only when the staff, managers and service users come together to define what this means for them that a shared vision of the future can evolve. It is often possible to build and sustain a coalition around this vision; this can then be shared with other stakeholders.

Examples from Manchester

Before 1982 all specialist services for learning-disabled people in Manchester were delivered by the local authority. In the 1970s social services provided hostels, two day centres and a small team of specialist social workers. There was also a large number of Mancunians living in hospitals in Lancashire and Cheshire. Some of these people had been placed before the war.

The resettlement programme – to return, over a number of years, Manchester people to the city – was a major incentive to joint working. The North Western Regional Health Authority and the North West Association of Social Services Authorities agreed the process and protocol of this resettlement programme. *The Model District Service* published by the regional health authority in 1982 endorsed and articulated 'ordinary life' principles; it was agreed by all constituent authorities and formed the basis of the resettlement agreement.

In 1982 the regional health authority allocated funding to district health authorities for them to establish community services for people with learning disabilities. Most districts, including the three Manchester health authorities, established multidisciplinary community teams. These staff – nurses, psychologists, occupational therapists, speech and language therapists and physiotherapists – and the newly formed social services department specialist teams of social workers and domiciliary carers had to establish a working relationship.

Joint problem-solving, particularly around the resettlement process, took time but created the basis for a shared vision – the essential building-block of joint working. The 'hard' services – day residential and domiciliary care – were still almost exclusively local authority-managed. Health professionals assessed and treated users and increasingly provided staff training. There were difficulties: the direct care staff often saw the health professionals as impractical visionaries providing a 'hit and run' service; and some health staff rejected much of the existing service as falling so far outside the ordinary life model that it would be pointless to attempt to redress it.

The joint problem-solving successes usually centred around individuals – both people living with their families and people who had returned to Manchester.

The resettlement programme initially developed local authority-managed networks of group houses. The model supported by both agencies pushed the local authority (which was keen to avoid a two-tier service) into a hostel closure programme and to move individuals into ordinary housing.

In South Manchester the community learning disability nurses were based with social work teams. Each group of staff still had its own manager, but this shared accommodation gave a strong base for improved working relations. A few therapists and a resettlement social worker were also based in a day centre. Interestingly, the community nurses appeared to have more contact with the social work team than with their colleagues in the therapy team.

In Central Manchester the health team was based in a day centre. They developed much good practice with colleagues providing day care but had less contact with the social work teams, until this collaboration was actively fostered by management in both organisations and the local authority hostel closure plans were developed. This latter development provided an opportunity to further develop cross-agency working. One of the newly set up staffed houses was managed by a clinical manager, employed and professionally supervised by the health service, but working as part of the social services dispersed residential network and managing a joint team of residential staff. This led to considerable gains for people who had previously presented intractable behavioural problems (see Chapter 12 on clinically managed social care).

A development with a similar goal was established at a day centre in the north of the city, where NHS therapy professionals coordinated the support and intervention programmes with service users with multiple disabilities (see Chapter 8 on day services).

In the mid- to late 1980s loose collaborative joint management groups were established in both North and Central Manchester. These tended to flourish in proportion to the commitment of the managers involved in them: the local authority in particular experienced frequent changes of managers in the relevant posts.

A major step forward in joint working in Manchester occurred in 1989 when a joint service manager was appointed to manage the health and social services staff in South Manchester. The appointment was to the local authority but partly recharged to the South Manchester Health Authority. This arrangement was mainly attributable to key senior staff in both organisations who were committed to a joint working model. At the time there was no coordinator for the health team in post, and the community nurses had experienced shared offices with the social work staff while the therapists had been based in a room in the Adult Training Centre for six years.

The arrangement was set up before the onset of the contract culture and survived for the next five years on the basis of an exchange of letters between the organisations. The joint service manager (South Manchester) brought the therapists to work in the social services offices along with the nurses. The process of creating a multidisciplinary team across two agencies began. This provided single access for health and social care in the south of the city. The filling of professional vacancies, and a more structured system of accountability for management staff, demonstrated to those staff who were more sceptical that there were immediate advantages to the new model. The hostel and housing networks benefited from a more structured approach and from the lessons learnt in managing much larger institutions.

It seemed that being able to direct services without having to pay continual, disproportionate attention to managing the boundaries of those services as well as the opportunity to focus the energy of staff from both agencies gave South Manchester a more flexible use of resources, a higher profile and some small successes that made a real impact on users' lives.

In 1993 the South Manchester Community Unit became a third-wave health trust. In 1994 it combined with the community units of Central Manchester Healthcare Trust and the North Manchester Healthcare Trust to be a city-wide fourth-wave trust, the Mancunian Community Health NHS Trust.

The learning disability service – jointly managed in South Manchester but separately managed in the rest of the city – had tracked the develop-

> **Example**
>
> A project in the special care unit of the day centre, which was led by therapy and nursing staff, seemed to ensure more constructive daytimes for these people. An alliance with a group of parents led to the local authority funding a new independent trust which managed a staffed group home for three people with major care needs.

ment of a city-wide community trust. The two social services managers, two health managers and joint managers had begun to meet regularly to plan future services.

The trust and the social services department, which was going through a management review, had incentives, in the form of management savings, to extend the joint management arrangement city-wide. The location of the joint management team within the new trust paved the way for any later movement of staff out of the authority. At that time, the social services department had real concerns about central government's commitment to forcing local authorities to relinquish their monopoly of service provision. The threat to the department's provider services of any extension of the 85 per cent rule, in which 85 per cent of transferred money from social security funding of residential services had to be spent in the independent sector, was clear to senior officers and members. The opportunity to transfer services in the future to an NHS trust with coterminous boundaries and a shared vision of community and health care was made easier by placing the management of the joint learning disability service with the trust.

Resources and further reading

Alter, C. and Hage, J. (1993), *Organizations Working Together*, Newbury Park, CA: Sage.

Burton, M. (1997), 'Learning disability: developing a definition', *Journal of Learning Disabilities*, 1 (1), 37–43.

Burton, M. and Kellaway, M. (1995), 'Specialisation without separation: combining health and social services provision for people with learning disabilities', *Health and Social Care in the Community*, 3 (4), 263–7.

Dluhy, M. (1990), *Building Coalitions in the Human Services*, Newbury Park, CA: Sage.

North Western Regional Health Authority (1982), *A Model District Service*, Manchester (available from NWTDT, Calderstones, Mitton Road, Walley, Lancashire, BB6 9PE).

Pettigrew, A., Ferlie, E. and McKie, L. (1992), *Shaping Strategic Change: Making*

Change in Large Organisations – The Case of the National Health Service, London: Sage.

Standish, S., Perry, C. and Palk, N. (1994), 'Scoring doubles', *Health Service Journal*, **104** (5240), 26–7.

2 Designing the organisation
Mark Burton and Mike Kellaway

Introduction

Every so often our organisations seem to reinvent themselves. They usually do this through structural reorganisations but, as we shall see, there are other ways of renewing and redesigning organisations so that they can most effectively serve their intended functions.

The evolving organisation

We can look at organisations in a variety of ways. One is to ask the question, 'How is control exerted?'. Over time, several models of organisational control have evolved:

- **Simple control.** Simple organisational control is based on coercive authority – the direct personal supervision of work, the 'hiring and firing' of interchangeable staff. An example might be a small proprietor-run catering business.
- **Technical control.** Here control is embedded in machine systems, so that machines dictate the pace of work; it is usually associated with worker isolation and deskilling. This is the model of the mass production factory.
- **Bureaucratic control.** This approach to control is based on the centralisation of power, the formalisation of work tasks and processes, specialisation and hierarchies of legitimated authority. Banks and the civil service are classical examples.

- **Professional control.** This is characterised by self-regulation and an emphasis on credentials required to practise. Professionals traditionally work semi-autonomously within the organisation. Legal firms, the churches and traditional universities are examples of organisations with strong professional control strategies.

No organisation is a pure form of one of these 'ideal types'; the different approaches generally co-exist and compete for dominance. Health and welfare services traditionally combine the professional and bureaucratic forms, with the professional strategy being stronger in health services and the bureaucratic form being stronger in local government.

From the 1970s onwards many organisational sectors have attempted to subdue professionalism through the use of bureaucratic control strategies. An example of this was the introduction of managerial approaches to the health service in three successive waves of reorganisation – in 1974 and 1982, and with the 'Griffiths' introduction of 'general management' from 1984.

Since the 1980s, however, 'post-bureaucratic' forms of organisational control have emerged. Post-bureaucracy is often associated with the New Right attack on the welfare state, although it is not necessarily a New Right concept or development. Some of its features, such as the decentralisation of operational control, first appeared in left-wing Labour-controlled local authorities. Others emerged simultaneously in societies with a more collectivist consensus than Britain (for example, Germany, Italy). However, in British health and welfare systems they appeared within a new right-wing government agenda in the following form:

- minimal government provision and the retreat of the state
- quasi-markets, where services are purchased on the behalf of users by others
- decentralisation of operational management: this can be internal, with, for example, the devolution of budgetary authority and control (within tight parameters) or external, where a service is provided by another organisation altogether
- the neutralisation or co-opting of traditional power and interest groups: hospital consultants become budget holding 'clinical directors', senior nurses are demoted and social workers administer the community care budget
- a rhetoric of emphasis on results, outcomes and quality
- a rhetoric of emphasis on the 'consumer' choice and consultation: this has often meant choice for some – 'assisted places', council house sales, shareholding

- a drive to reduce public expenditure through efficiency savings, cash-limited budgets, eligibility criteria and outright cuts but within the constraints of political possibility: for example, the public still has a high regard for the NHS.

The above developments have been mirrored in learning disability services, with a progression from its origins rooted in philanthropy and the Victorian Poor Law, via the public service model of health and social services, to the present emerging picture whose post-bureaucratic characteristics appear to be:

- the residual nature of local government provision, illustrated by the '85 per cent rule' which requires 85 per cent of the Special Transitional Grant (transferred from the social security budget to the local authority for community care) has to be spent outside the authority in the independent sector: this is consistent with the notion of the 'enabling' but not 'providing' public authority
- emphasis on consumer power, but chiefly through the 'exit' mechanism of the market, rather than through the 'voice' channels of advocacy and the political process
- increasing decentralisation of decision-making within the organisation
- 'softer' organisational boundaries – for example, with staff employed by one organisation (say, a NHS trust) working within the provision of another organisation (such as an independent sector or social services-run home)
- increasing emphasis on quality, effectiveness and outcomes, with the clear aim that this must be grounded in the living experiences of the people with learning disabilities themselves
- the existence of a user voice, which is slowly increasing in confidence and strength, together with an increased sophistication about how to read the views and interests of people with less obvious means of communication
- continuing pressure for efficiency in service provision and repeated 'cut and come again' budgetary reductions.

It is difficult to say how much all of the above developments are a result of the 'post-bureaucratic shift', but that has been the context which has enabled and encouraged these changes, often in conjunction with other movements and emphases.

During this period social services departments have veered between specialism and genericism, function versus locality, and vertical versus horizontal integration, as organising principles. Some of these swings also reflect the 'long-wave' changes in organisational theory and social policy identified above.

Key issues

In deciding how to organise a service there are some key issues to identify and address.

Is a change necessary?

Changing the structure of an organisation is not necessarily the best way to improve performance. We believe that, in some circumstances, real gains can be made from altering structures – for example, by focusing management effort more effectively on manageable chunks of the service or by creating 'self fertilising' work groups from staff with different skills, knowledge, and experience. But consider carefully whether, in your case, more might be gained by making changes in something other than structure (examples include staff knowledge, work practices and processes, systems for organising and managing work and information, culture, vision, philosophy and relationships with other parts of the service system). The old adage, 'If it isn't broken, don't try to fix it' is relevant here.

Building-blocks

It is tempting to design the organisation from the 'top down', reflecting existing organisational divisions and ways of organising, rather than asking the question:

What organisational design will best support what the service is trying to achieve?

An alternative approach is to establish from the outset the building-blocks of the service. The key question, then, is:

What are the basic elements of the service, from which the organisation can be built up?

One way of thinking about this is in terms of the 'viable' or potentially autonomous elements of the service. There is no one correct way of defining this: in a rural service with a dispersed population it makes sense to think in terms of geographical units, while in an urban service functional specialisation (by type of service) probably makes more sense. We will return to this question.

Having identified the building-blocks (for example, three dispersed supported housing networks, two community teams, three day services), the next question is:

How should these building-blocks be put together managerially?

In the above example, three divisions based on supported housing, services to families and professional services, and day services might make sense. Having established these relatively autonomous divisions it must then be considered how they will be coordinated as a whole, how they will relate to one another and how relations will be managed with their environments. Broadly, we advise that each unit has the managerial authority to manage its own relationships within clear parameters. This then frees the overall management to focus on the more complex managerial tasks, such as planning and development, industrial relations, quality issues including complaints, training, and management of relationships with other organisations including commissioners of services. In setting up the organisation in this way it is important to check that each level is as self-sufficient as possible to conduct its own business and that information flows (which include personal contact) can take place in a way that makes sure that each element of the service is equipped for its defined management tasks. Some resources for organisational design are listed at the end of the chapter.

Functional versus geographical

This distinction was made above in the previous section. To aid your analysis of which approach is more suitable consider the following questions:

1 Does the service have to be delivered in a way that is sensitive to local community differences? We suspect that the answer is usually 'Yes'.
2 Does this mean that all services have to be managed together, locally, or can a functional division (for example, all the supported living networks) have an overall management, with each unit (that is, each network) being managed locally?
3 Is there anything to be gained by managing more than one type of service together on a local basis (for example, managing the community domiciliary service together with the dispersed residential service, thereby allowing flexibility of staffing)? Is there likely to be a problem

with this – for example, will one element of the service pull resources too easily from another, because there is no 'buffer' between them?

4   Is there anything which makes it appropriate to manage all services of one type together – for example a big change agenda, such as the need to improve standards across all day services, at least while the change is being implemented?

Central versus local management and control

All organisations balance local and central management control in some way. How will you balance the need for an overall consistent approach with the need for decision-making as near as possible to the point-of-service delivery? To help decide, consider the following questions:

1   What organisational tasks have to be carried out? These may include budget-setting, expenditure, recruitment, handling complaints, discipline, grievances, staff development, supervision of practice, planning, and managing relations with the wider organisation, other organisations and the public.

2   Which of these are best done locally, and which require a system overview?

3   What are the organisation's constraints on such tasks as formulating local policies, devolving budgets and so on?

4   What is the capacity of managers at each level to handle these tasks? It might be a feasible medium-term goal to decentralise more decision-making, once local managers have been briefed, trained, and support systems for them set up.

Accountability to the organisation(s)

The operation of the service must be accountable, ultimately to the highest level of the organisation, but how is this to be achieved? How will the people who are supposed to be responsible for the service know what it is actually doing? How can they find out without disrupting the service itself (for example, by having such demands for information that too much time is taken away from service provision, or by interfering so much in local decisions that staff and junior managers feel constantly watched, not trusted, and powerless)? What systems and methods of supervision and audit will be used, and who will be responsible for them?

Management support functions

To run an effective organisation, a variety of 'management support functions' must be served. These are the functions that are not concerned with service delivery or the management of the service itself, but are necessary for management to draw upon to work effectively. They include:

- personnel, including recruitment
- administration and clerical support
- finance, including accounting, budgeting, and payroll services
- information services
- supplies
- estates and building management
- legal services
- contract management.

Decisions have to be taken about how these functions will be served. The decisions are likely to be made by higher levels of the organisation, but there may be some scope for choice of arrangements. Some organisations centralise these functions more than others, and overcentralisation (for example, holding all budgets centrally, being unable to source anything without reference to a supplies department) can impair organisational effectiveness. It is also possible to have many of these functions served at the level of service management, thereby distracting managers from the core purposes of the service – for example, managers have to struggle with tax issues rather than manage the care and support provided to service users. Some of these functions are increasingly likely to be provided outside the organisation itself.

Development and quality

Development and quality are important functions for the organisation's future survival. There is a dilemma regarding whether, and to what extent, these should be separate functions or functions that are part of everybody's work. It is a matter of balance: if development and quality are only considered by a centralised department, which is insulated from the provision of service, it is likely to generate strategies and practices that are irrelevant to the service. At the other extreme, if these functions are just taken to be everyone's business, they are likely to be given a low priority.

The decision to be made, then, is about how the processes of development and quality improvement can be *led*, but in a way that *involves* people who have an intimate knowledge of the provision of the service (which does not just mean managers and staff). In a small organisation it will not usually be possible to do more than identify a 'lead responsibility' for work on quality. A large organisation might have one or more development specialists. In both cases, the work of these quality and development leaders needs to be integrated into both the work of managing the service and its delivery. Part IV, 'Safeguarding Quality', illustrates some strategies for this task.

Perceptions and anxieties

It is more likely that a reorganisation of one or more services is envisaged rather than the creation of an entirely new service. Nevertheless, however good your design, people will have their own perceptions and anxieties about what you are doing. These concerns will primarily centre around what they might lose – for example:

- their job
- control over their work
- job satisfaction
- good working relationships
- links and support with others in their line of work
- status and influence
- familiarity with their work, clients, practices, neighbourhoods.

Other concerns will have to do with what their clients might lose:

- resources
- commitment
- understanding
- familiarity

Familiarity appears in both the above lists, and it is a key issue in change: people tend to fear – or at least distrust – the unknown. Even if the change is worthwhile, many will find it unsettling. In most of our organisations there is a legacy of reorganisation that has achieved little: why should people believe your reorganisation is going to be any different?

These perceptions and anxieties must be worked with, both to support staff, service users and their allies during an unsettling period and to ensure the continuity of the service itself. If people feel badly treated, that their interests and concerns are not recognised, then they are likely to perform badly or leave. While some staff turnover is to be expected, it should be monitored during periods of change.

Practical guidance

Communication

Communication within each agency and with all stakeholders is critical to the success of any attempt to redesign an organisation. For learning disability services the following are crucial.

- **Purchasers or commissioners of services.** Provider services do need to ensure that their proposed organisational arrangements and models of service delivery are consistent with the purchasers' plans. A regular forum for communication is valuable in creating a shared strategy and an environment with 'few nasty surprises'.
- **Service users and their allies.** It is often difficult to consult meaningfully with users and their families about the reorganisation of services, particularly if it is a global, rather than single-unit, reorganisation. However, users and their families tend to be concerned with the outcome of reorganisation, and this can be chastening for managers who can become overabsorbed in the mechanics of the service (process and structure) and neglect to think through whether and how such changes will affect people who rely on it. It is often more effective to communicate proposals (more than one option!) to representative groups than try to work from a 'blank piece of paper'.
- **Staff.** Particularly where services are merging (as in the creation of a Joint Service or interorganisational management agreement) there is a need to involve staff and their representatives. There may, for example, be concern that existing terms and conditions, or disciplinary and grievance procedures, will not be honoured (although such matters are governed by EU legislation on 'Transfer of Undertakings'). Staff may fear that the present phase of reorganisation (for example, a joint management arrangement) could be a 'slippery slope' to more radical changes, such as a full transfer of employment. It is worth considering formal communication systems such as team briefings or even a 'rumour hotline' so that staff can check what they may have heard directly with a senior person.

All the above involve two-way communication – not just 'telling' but also listening and adapting. Nobody – not even those charged with leadership and management roles – has a monopoly on information or wisdom.

Structure

As indicated above, it is essential to be clear about the basic building-blocks/functions which will underpin the organisation of the service. There will inevitably be constraints on the extent and costs of the management structure, but it is only when there is clarity about the basis of the service that the structure can be planned.

In deciding between functional or geographical models it may be worth considering a combination of the two approaches.

Consider carefully spans of control. Managers become ineffective if they have too many staff to support, lead and manage.

It is also important to avoid being steered by precedents: these will have often grown incrementally under circumstances that no longer exist, and will have little to commend them. Figure 2.1 shows the pattern of responsibilities in one social services department which used vertical organisation for client groups and geographical area teams for fieldwork. In the figure, these vertical lines of function and horizontal lines of user group required such good communication and management skills to administer that they proved ineffective.

	Assistant Director: Residential	Assistant Director: Domiciliary	Assistant Director: fieldwork
Children and families	X	X	X
Services to older people	X	X	X
Mental health	X	X	X
Learning disability	X	X	X

Figure 2.1   Resulting pattern of responsibilities from using both vertical and geographical organisational structures

The eventual management structure will also be affected by the administrative support available. It is often at reorganisation that the crucial role of administration and secretarial support is recognised.

Skills

In keeping with the principle of making each building-block of the service as self-sufficient as possible, it is worth considering carefully the blend of skills that will be available within each staff team – including the management teams. For example, are there people with strengths in the following areas?

- Leading
- Negotiating
- Innovating
- Developing
- Maintaining
- Finishing.

All will need to be team players as the task of 'selling' the effectiveness of the new working arrangements will require not only managers, but also staff, to speak with 'one voice' on core issues. Much careful work can be undone by someone breaking ranks and making public statements based on misunderstanding or idiosyncratic beliefs: such ideas should not be suppressed, but articulated and debated at the appropriate time and place, (such as in team meetings).

Control versus participation

Many restructuring organisations find that making the centralisation of control the first task helps ensure that the organisation has a consistent shared vision and approach to service delivery. The more radical the re-structure, the more new policies, procedures, and guidelines on practice will 'rush from the press'. This can understandably feel like an over-bureaucratising of the service: gradually moving to a participative model of management is possible although the suspicions of staff that senior management is still 'pulling the strings' takes a while to shift.

There is an important balancing act between driving the new service into place and being prepared to be flexible and responsive in implementation. Having a management team that has worked together (even from separate divisions or organisations as was the case in Manchester) can certainly help in the process.

An example from Manchester: setting up the Joint Learning Disability Service

In 1993 the 'shadow' Mancunian Community Health NHS Trust and the social services department made a decision in principle to establish a jointly managed learning disability service. Three main benefits were envisaged, and these became cornerstones in designing the new organisation:

1   It would provide a seamless service. People with learning disabilities and their families would not have to determine whether their need is for social or health support. There would be a common and open referral system through a single access point for all services provided.
2   Whether employed by the health service or social services, all staff in each part of the service would report to a single manager. This would help ensure the focus, impetus and authority to effect change.
3   'Specialisation without separation' was the aim. This would allow the specialisation of functions without separation into different services and allow integration of specialist skills within the support systems for people living ordinary lives in the community. This would not only help create a shared responsibility and shared understanding of priorities but would also help ensure that collaboration took place and was followed through (for example, when a care manager requested a health service employee to carry out an assessment, or when a health employee made recommendations to social services staff regarding appropriate ways of supporting a person's special needs).

The managers of the existing services provided by three health service trusts and one social services department met on a monthly basis throughout 1993. These meetings focused initially on the collaborative shared management of the existing services (including redevelopment from hostels, people requiring complex supports to remain at home, increasing professional input to people using day services and so on), but increasingly became concerned with the planning of the new Joint Service.

At the end of 1993 the Social Services Committee requested assurances that the lack of direct political accountability of the new NHS Trust to the people of Manchester could be overcome. The chief executive of the Mancunian Community Health NHS Trust then spoke to the members of the Social Services Committee. Subsequently, agreement to proceed to the creation of a city-wide Joint Learning Disability Service was given at the trust board meeting and Social Services Committee meeting in January 1994.

The Joint Service Managers' Group, which already met monthly, was established as a task group. It prepared an audit of the current service, staff, budgets, and office and equipment resources. It was understood that the reconfigured service should demonstrate an equity of provision across the city: what was available in Harpurhey should also be available in Moss Side and Wythenshawe.

At that time, the NHS and Community Care Act was being implemented, and the social services department was developing the purchaser–provider split in its community care division. The embryo Joint Service would be a provider service managing domiciliary and residential care services and community health staff who provided health care. The Social Services Committee needed reassurance that the standards and quality of both the Joint Service and the growing number of independent providers would be monitored. Since 1990 the existing social services resettlement project manager had been purchasing services from the independent sector, for people returning to the city from large hospitals. Since this small team had experience in negotiating contracts and monitoring quality, it was proposed it be expanded into a purchasing team, purchasing all residential and domiciliary services for people with learning disabilities. It would also monitor the Joint Service.

Another key issue was the situation of social workers/care managers. Early purist dogma about the purchaser–provider split would have them located on the purchasing side. Their principal role was to assess, plan and review support arrangements (or 'care packages' in the strange jargon of these times) for individual people. Increasingly, such supports were being provided by the independent sector. However, learning-disabled people and their families did not fit easily into the 'assess–place–monitor' model of care management, since their circumstances and needs changed regularly and had to be maintained over many years. The interwoven supports included day occupation, respite, leisure opportunities, skill development and therapy, employment and health care. The old social work role had been largely abandoned by social workers for older people as they became care managers under the changes brought about by the NHS and Community Care Act. That role, which included elements of direct provision, service coordination, monitoring and intervention, negotiation and advocacy, was still a critical ingredient of support for people with learning disabilities. This user group would not be served well by the 'assess and place' model. A significant number of people lived independently only because a social worker or care manager organised their support on a daily and weekly basis. A large and increasing number of people needed a combination of health and social support and care. It was realised that a purist model of care management as purchasing could result in a split between the health and social services practitioners.

To resolve these issues it was agreed that the balance of the social worker/ care managers who remained after a number were allocated to the purchasing team and a newly created disabled children's team would be located within the Joint Service. Day services were specifically excluded from consideration by the Joint Service Managers' Group. The social services department decided to keep this under its direct control and within a broader umbrella that included employment support services. The task group commented that at least that part of day services which related to people with more complex needs would benefit considerably by being part of a joint service.

The task group identified the basic building-blocks of the service. In one version these were:

1 home support (networks and relatively high intensity domiciliary support – for example more than 15 hours per week)
2 daytime support (day care)*
3 technical support (training/therapy/specialised assessment/intervention/behavioural management)
4 family support (practical input to people and their families)
5 service development and integration (quality improvement, planning, marketing, training and so on)
6 management support (accountancy, personnel – provided corporately – secretarial/admin.).

A variety of issues were considered before defining the options for structuring the management of these services. The following questions were asked.

1 How close to the user/locality can we organise the various service functions – what is smallest viable service building-block?
2 What are the sources of conflict/oscillation? In other words, what will have to be managed in order for these building-blocks to continue functioning effectively?
3 What kind of sensors does the service need, at each level – to detect

   – threats to, and opportunities for, sustainability/effectiveness/efficiency
   – overseeing of system/service remit/goals
   – innovation inside/outside

4 What will be the goals of this organisation?

* Daytime support was included in the early discussions since there were strong arguments for its inclusion in the Joint Service.

5   How will detection of changes be used to steer and adjust the system? In other words, what arrangements are there for decision-making and development? What elements are needed in the decision-making parts?
6   How will resources be allocated to/among constituent system parts?

- What safeguards the accuracy/justness of this resource bargaining
- How will performance be measured?
- What does this imply for the knowledge/skills/capacity of the overall (higher) management of the (learning disability) service?

7   What are our assumptions about the nature of task/organisations/people?
8   What works well now?

In addition, it was recognised that someone has to (or some people have to):

- manage the basic blocks of the service day-to-day
- deputise for these day-to-day managers
- manage these managers
- allocate resources (and establish rules, principles, measures for doing so)
- monitor resource usage
- sense changes in the environment
- sense changes in the service itself
- set standards
- question and develop practices
- arrange training at all levels
- monitor practices and standards
- act on information so collected
- look ahead
- type the letters, reports, minutes and so on
- acquire and defend the service's resources
- take overall responsibility
- monitor staff performance
- investigate complaints, grievances and so on
- discipline staff and so on
- manage the boundaries with other services.

These questions, once brought to the surface, could help in choosing among options for structuring the new service although in the time available, not every issue could be covered in sufficient detail. The task group proposed a functional model with geographical divisions, and this was accepted, with some amendments, by the director of social services and chief executive of the trust. The model had the following elements:

1   A head of service had already been specified.
2   A residential manager would be responsible for the eight network teams supporting people living in dispersed housing, a further network and an NHS house providing respite care. It was argued that these services, some of which had significant problems at that time, ought to be managed centrally in order to ensure a consistent approach to quality and accountability.
3   The management resources available determined that there would be four community learning disability teams (CLDTs). On the basis of ward divisions, the city could be divided into four localities of 100 000 to 110 000. Each CLDT would have a manager. Initially there was not sufficient funding for four CLDT managers, and the social services department agreed to pay for the temporary upgrading of a member of staff: The Joint Service would make sufficient savings to fund the post within the first year. There would be two area managers, each responsible for two CLDTs as well as some of the other functions that had been identified. In one management model proposed, the Joint Service had a business manager responsible for business planning, administrative support, finance, information, marketing and contracting and complaints: in the end, these responsibilities were shared among the management team. However, such a post would have been an asset during the period of establishing the Joint Service.
4   Subsequent to the task group's recommendations, the post of head of development and clinical services was created to provide a clinical lead while encompassing quality and development. The post-holder also had responsibility for services to people presenting behavioural challenges. One of his first tasks was to resolve professional leadership within the single management model. Another early task was to interweave the existing additional support teams (for people with challenging behaviour) into the CLDTs. The resolution of these issues is described elsewhere.

The resulting structure of the service is shown in Figures 2.1 and 2.2.

Reconfiguring the service

The creation of the CLDTs is discussed in detail in Chapter 3. The guiding principle of equity of service required the movement of staff from their current locations to the four new teams. Each member of staff was invited

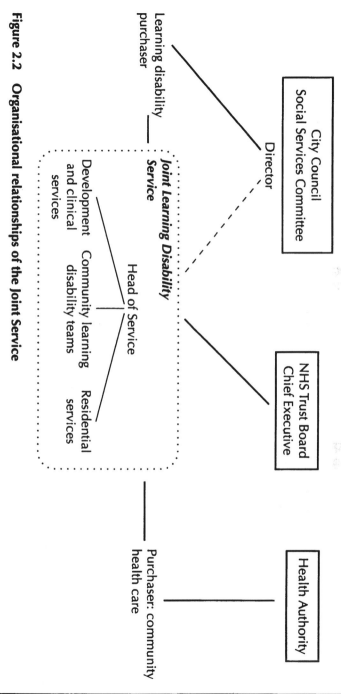

Figure 2.2   Organisational relationships of the Joint Service

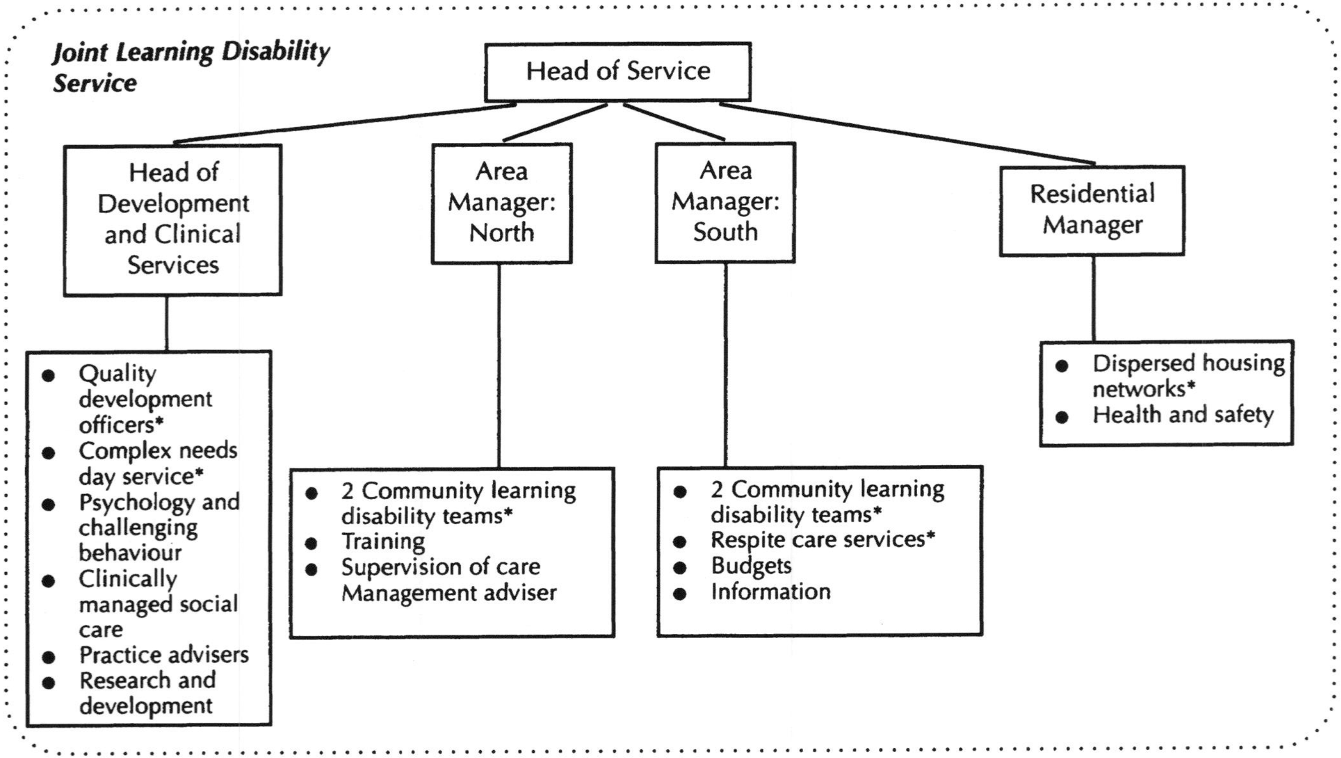

Joint Learning Disability Service

Head of Service

Head of Development and Clinical Services
- Quality development officers*
- Complex needs day service*
- Psychology and challenging behaviour
- Clinically managed social care
- Practice advisers
- Research and development

Area Manager: North
- 2 Community learning disability teams*
- Training
- Supervision of care
- Management adviser

Area Manager: South
- 2 Community learning disability teams*
- Respite care services*
- Budgets
- Information

Residential Manager
- Dispersed housing networks*
- Health and safety

* Indicates line management responsibilities.

Figure 2.3   Current structure of the Joint Learning Disability Service

to state their first, second and third preferences: over 85 per cent of staff received their first or second choice. Some negotiation was possible for those who were dissatisfied with the initial outcome of this process.

The creation of a Joint Service was considerably eased by the commitment of senior officers and the chairs of the trust board and Social Services Committee. The fact that the health and social services learning disability managers had worked together over many years made it possible to share a vision of how services could look within a joint management arrangement. The commitment of staff to improve services and the cooperation of trade unions were also crucial to its success.

Resources and further reading

Beer, S. (1985), *Diagnosing the System for Organisation*, Chichester: Wiley.
  The approach to designing organisational structures is based loosely on 'Viable System Diagnosis', a cybernetic model developed by this author.
Flood, R.L. (1995), *Solving Problem Solving: A Potent Force for Effective Management*, Chichester: Wiley.
  Explains VSD in more accessible terms, within the context of a variety of methods for management problem-solving.
Other material worth looking at is as follows.
Clegg, S. (1981), 'Organisation and control', *Administrative Science Quarterly* **26**, 545–62.
Hoggett, P. (1991), 'A new management in the public sector?', *Policy and Politics* **19** (4), 243–56.
Mintzberg, H. (1983), *Structure in Fives: Designing Effective Organisations*, Englewood Cliffs, NJ: Prentice-Hall.
The Audit Commission (1996), *Form Follows Function: Changing Management Structures in the NHS and Local Government*, ISBN 1 86240 000 8.

Part II

Equipping, Supporting and Leading Staff

Introduction

Services for people with learning disabilities are very 'staff-intensive'; they depend on people rather than buildings and equipment. Indeed, perhaps the most significant change over the last 15 years has been to convert resources that were not used in the direct support of people (especially buildings, ancillary staff) into staff who work closely with people in ordinary community settings.

How good are services at equipping, supporting and leading all these staff? What issues must be tackled, and what do we know about what works? Equipping, supporting and leading staff can be divided into the following areas:

- definition of role and tasks
- policies and procedures
- supervision and appraisal
- management visibility
- training and staff development
- problem-solving with staff.

The following four chapters explore these issues through the experience of setting up and managing community learning disability teams (CLDTs), managing dispersed housing networks, setting up a joint training strategy, and policies and procedures respectively. The best approach to follow will depend on three factors:

1 *The skills, knowledge, experience and confidence of the staff.* Have they formal training or a qualification in this work? How much learning have they done on (and from) the job? How wide a range of experience do

they have (including experience from other parts of their life, such as running a household)? Does all this mean that they are confident in dealing with the situations that are likely to arise?

2 *The situation in which they work.* Are they working in a setting with management or more experienced staff present, or are they working in situations that are relatively 'invisible' to those who could provide guidance?

3 *The nature of the work.* How difficult is the work? How predictable are the demands of the work – how flexible will staff have to be in their approach and how much discretion and judgement do they have to use? How much skill, knowledge and experience is needed? How stressful is the work – do the pressures come in bursts, or are they fairly constant over time?

In the case of the CLDTs and housing networks the pattern is as shown in Table II.1. The pattern illustrated in the table has led to rather different approaches in the two divisions of the service, although there are strategies in common (such as building strong teams with a shared vision) which permeate the entire service.

Chapter 5, 'Joint Training' identifies the characteristics of a strategy relevant to all sectors and illustrates this in relation to the Manchester experience.

Finally, Chapter 6, on policies, analyses the functions of policies, gives a guide to their production, and illustrates this by way of an example.

Table II.1   Working patterns of CLDTs and housing networks

Service	Staff characteristics	Work situation	Nature of work
CLDT	50% professionally qualified: few over 40, some newly qualified; others highly experienced. 50% unqualified, wide age range, varying length of service.	Community settings including service users' homes and other settings. Mostly 'invisible' because so dispersed. Some coworking (for example, across disciplines).	High levels of discretion and judgement. Wide variation in task demands and stress. (Some CLDT staff define tasks to be carried out by others.)
Housing networks	Mostly unqualified. Wide range of backgrounds including university graduates, ex-ancillary staff, staff with experience of other care settings.	Mostly in ordinary houses with tenants in groups of up to four. May be working alone for long periods (except at handovers, or in settings with higher levels of user need). Will also be supporting tenants in ordinary community settings (for example, leisure facilities, shops).	A core of prescribed and predictable tasks concerned with tenant and household care. Moderate levels of discretion and judgement. Wide variation in task demands and stress.

3 Leading and directing staff in community teams: tales of the unexpected

Maxine Martin and Bernie Gibbins, with Christine Adcock

Introduction

The 'vision' for joint working emerged against the backdrop of the National Health Service and Community Care Act 1990, the increase in accountability, 'consumer market choice' and pressure to reduce staff. At this point, the consideration of staff morale was fundamental. The way staff are equipped, supported, maintained and encouraged to develop through this minefield of change is crucial.

To enable staff to move forward by rebuilding and developing, it may be necessary to include a process of review of past experience and challenge the traditional 'we've always done it this way' attitude. Preconceptions around roles/worker expectation and service provision have to be addressed. A time of change permits the re-evaluation of what has become custom and practice.

A fundamental consideration in this has to be to include and value each individual member of staff. Theories on how we cope with change identify various possible responses since people cope with change in many different ways. When organisations restructure, large numbers of people experience and react to this disruption simultaneously. A manager faced with this situation needs a variety of skills (many of which are not at all obvious) in order to lead their staff along the path being taken by the organisation. Managers themselves also need to be supported if they are to be effective; they also need a shared vision of the new organisation.

Collaboration depends on cooperation rather than alienation, and clear and consistent messages about the negotiable and non-negotiable aspects of the changes.

The manager will require a variety of attributes, which can be listed as follows:

- honesty
- openness
- empathy
- the ability to identify good practice
- observation and interpretation skills
- clarity of direction
- an awareness of service objectives
- the ability to demonstrate positive leadership
- accessibility and awareness of day-to-day issues
- a non-confrontational approach to staff resistance
- an awareness of, and ability to identify, staff training needs
- the ability to support staff positively in their approaches and attitudes to developing their own skills
- mediation and negotiation skills both within the team and with other elements of the service and external organisations
- the ability to assist staff in recognising wider, local and national, issues which create the necessity for change – for example, legislation
- good receptive listening skills directed towards other issues which may be shaping staff effectiveness – for example, personal home issues
- a recognition of own strengths and weaknesses.

Facing the change

The scenario

In April 1994 not only were the legislative and policy changes working their way through to service delivery but, in Manchester, the Joint Service had just reconfigured its inherited field services into four joint community learning disability teams (see Chapter 2). A key principle at this point was to ensure the maintenance of the existing service provision, whilst preparing it for change. The manager needed a good understanding of service users' needs, the short- and long-term aims of the organisation, and the interests, concerns and capabilities of the staff.

The action

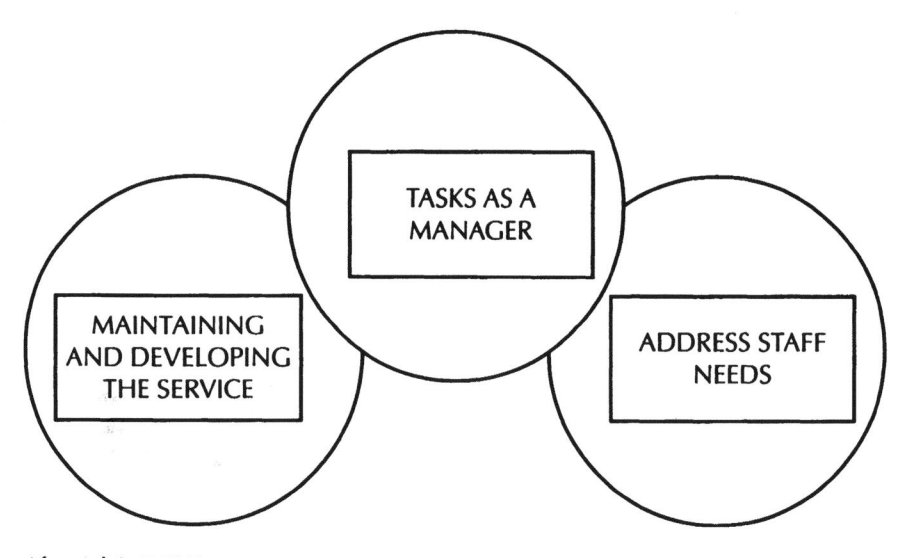

After Adair (1983)

Figure 3.1 Summary of team manager's areas of action

We identified a series of questions that enabled the managers to gain a clearer picture of the boundaries of their task:

- What does the client need?
- What does the organisation expect/demand?
- What does the legislation require?
- What skills do the staff have?
- At what stage are the staff in coping with the change, and what do they need to be able to move on positively?
- What 'history' – hopes, dreams, prejudices, preconceived ideas, doubts, fears, knowledge, skills and experience – have the staff brought with them?
- What 'bridges' need to be built in the new structure?
- What 'walls' need to be 'demolished' to enhance the service?
- What are the team's strengths and weaknesses?
- What skills do I have as a manager and what help/support do I need? Who tells me or gives me sensible non-partisan feedback?
- How much control should I take at this point?
- How do I demonstrate my leadership?

- How much responsibility is within my control and how much is the responsibility of the wider organisation?
- Where do I start and finish as a manager?

Figure 3.1 summarises the action.

Reaction to change

It was easy to recognise in individuals the responses to change that are often highlighted in theories on change management (for example, Adair, 1983; Plant, 1987):

- **Denial**. This is the proverbial 'ostrich syndrome' – 'If I keep my head down (in the sand) and get on with my job, everything will stay the same and the "changes" will go away' or 'There is no change – it's a fallacy. Nothing is going to change anyway.'
- **Resistance and anger**. 'I'll fight you all the way.'
- **Anxiety and personalisation**. 'They're out to get me. Why is this happening? I can't do my work and cope with all of this.'
- **Insecurity**. 'They're doing this to cut costs … will my job be the next to go?'
- **Loss**. 'My job is going to change … I may have to move to another room or building, or change my working relationships.'

At this point the manager had to realise that some of these reactions were based in reality. Yes, you may have to move to a different building. Yes, you may have to learn new skills. Yes, you may have to take on roles that you had previously resisted. It was crucial to be honest – clouding change with confused messages only increases anxiety and leads to more negative responses.

Balance of control

There is a fine line between too much control and too little. There are probably no clear directions that can be given, except to know yourself and get to know your staff. Clarify the organisation's expectations, and find your allies. What can you afford to delegate and what must you deal with yourself?

Certain staff within the service had additional anxieties that compounded their needs for support and direction. The context in which restructuring takes place will often impact more on some jobs than on others. These staff will feel particularly vulnerable and exposed. In 1993–94 the social services department was undergoing fundamental changes driven by the NHS and Community Care Act, which required the development of a split between purchasing and provision. Social workers metamorphosed into care managers overnight. In the midst of the creation of a joint service the social work staff had to rethink and retrain to fulfil a new role.

Maintaining provision during change

Whilst the scenery and scripts are being altered ... 'the show must go on'.

Service provision was maintained as consistently as possible due to the shared value base of 'ordinary life principles' held at all levels by both health and social services staff. This was further supported by ensuring maximum communication to both staff and users via consultation and information meetings.

Throughout this process it was crucial for team managers to have open, two-way channels of communication with more senior management. The manager needed to know:

- where the service stood at that time
- where the service was expected to be in the short-term
- what the longer-term future might look like
- which aspects would be helpful to the future
- which aspects would present obstacles to the future.

Practical guidance

Minimise rumour and maximise fact

During times of uncertainty and change, rumours can spread and cause misunderstanding, exerting a malign effect on morale and cooperation. Formal methods for briefing people on changes are therefore important. In Manchester, the 'team brief' system for informing all staff of news and developments was one way of ensuring that everyone at least had access to the 'official story'.

Get to know the staff

In Manchester, this was done both formally through supervision (job consultation) and less formally through discussions, meetings and observation.

Establish a team structure

Begin a routine which will support a sense of security for the staff – that is, set up meetings, structures, define areas of responsibility and so on. This enables the staff to begin to acknowledge and reaffirm their individual roles within the evolving service structure.

Phase in new ideas ... carefully

A 'bull in a china shop' approach does not work and only increases staff anxiety. New ideas and structures can be tried and evaluated; some will be discarded. There is a need for honesty about what decisions are the prerogative of management and which can best be made by consensus.

Traditions are important for us all – recognising when these need to change or new patterns need to be established is important. In Manchester, the enthusiasm and shared vision of the managers fuelled positive proposals for change.

Bring the team together

Team-building exercises are vital for coping with change. In Manchester, each team depending on personalities and structure, used a variety of methods to achieve this. An example of the agenda for one such session contained:

1 *Views on change.* This was a flipchart exercise, 'What does change mean to you?'.
2 *Sharing experiences.* This raised the issue that we are all facing change and that change has been forced on us. An exercise, 'How do you cope with change outside of work?' involved identifying a change that had happened at home, what the person did and how they felt afterwards.
3 *Marking change.* Celebration of success and 'good news' stories were described to lead people into recognising that they needed to move on from where they were previously and help them develop the new 'joint' teams.
4 *Theory.* Theoretical perspectives on change, including 'force field analysis' were discussed and information on understanding and managing change (see 'References and Resources', p. 57) were made available.

As the staff worked through this agenda, the manager helped them translate it into what the team was feeling and what it needed to do to get through the difficulties. In the early days this helped the staff find mutual support. They realised that they were all facing change and, rather than withdraw into 'small groups' and establish a 'siege mentality', they were able to begin to support each other.

It was helpful to build in reflective sessions outside of usual business meetings. These are not easy to get commitment for as there are always many pressing jobs to be done, but the bringing and sharing of food helped. Food can be a wonderful team-building asset!

By this stage, the team manager should have clearly identified him or herself as the leader of the group. The team manager has to establish an understanding that he or she can and will exercise authority, but will do so in a fair, principled and accountable manner. A culture of openness helps here. The leader has a clear duty to enable team members to begin to clarify and develop their role and to understand the roles of others.

Further team exercises can focus on this issue in greater depth; however, it is an important ongoing daily process in supporting and equipping staff in order to create an effective service.

Build shared working

As regularly as possible encourage shared working, especially between those from different backgrounds and disciplines to build a common culture and avoid 'balkanisation' into professional enclaves. In Manchester, for example, all new referrals were jointly assessed by a care manager and nurse: this fostered mutual understanding as well as enhancing assessment practice in both groups.

Regular appraisal

The team manager needs to be constantly aware of how the current situation (at any point in time) relates to future goals and should take corrective action where necessary. Without this reflective stance the whole service can drift into a set of customs and practices that have their origins and rationales in one phase of the service's development but which become increasingly inappropriate as services change and the new service matures.

Support for the manager

As a manager you may have the skills and personality, but you definitely need support from those who understand your position.

In Manchester, regular meetings with peers – that is, other team managers – frequent contact, regular checking out and brainstorming sessions and sharing skills all helped to increase confidence and build support. It is important to ensure that support is sufficiently challenging and critical: if you are getting something wrong who will tell you? It can help to establish a safe, but honest, means of obtaining feedback: in our experience people tend to be kind and considerate when they do this, and in a well run team there should be few surprises. Such an approach also helps staff feel that they are listened to and taken seriously.

Developing and encouraging new ways of working

Several interlocking approaches were used to improve and develop working practices in the development of the Manchester Joint Service.

Ownership

Many of the new ideas in the service have to go through a process of trial and error, but staff need to be positive about change and take an active part in bringing it about. The manager's role of delegating responsibility to team members helps staff to have a sense of ownership in changing practices to meet the needs of both the service user and the organisation. Moreover, on some issues, leadership from peers can be more effective than that from managers.

Throughout these moves, the service recognised that good practice, valuable skills and service enhancement would be best served by ensuring that staff felt well supported and clear about their future direction.

Support and supervision

At this point the Joint Service needed to look at how this support would be provided – there were clearly two levels, managerial and professional.

It was agreed that managerial support would be provided by the team managers who were responsible for allocating resources. This took the form of regular job consultation meetings which covered the following issues:

- Housekeeping
  - leave
  - mileage.
- Operational
  - workload
  - case coordination

- capacity
- resources.

- Development

  - general training
  - project work in the team.

Outside of these formal meetings, the team managers created and encouraged an open-door environment so that team members could access the manager when and as needed.

The Joint Service was also able to maintain and extend the clinical supervision structures that were already in place. The larger scale of the service (now city-wide) helped in this, reducing professional isolation. All professional staff have a professional supervisor and, for each profession, the senior supervisor is the practice adviser for that discipline, with responsibilities to advise both their professional colleagues and management. Professional supervision would focus on such issues as:

- Professional development

  - competencies/skills needed
  - specialist training
  - trust-wide professional issues.

- Practice

  - work methods
  - new practice developments
  - grade/workload match
  - review of cases (more complex ones with more experienced staff).

This was not an entirely new initiative for the health professionals but it could have left the social services care managers feeling isolated as a professional group. The Joint Service negotiated an additional payment for one of the care managers so that they could take on a similar role to their senior health colleagues. Practice advisers, in turn, are professionally supported by senior colleagues outside the Joint Service to ensure that they are in tune with local and national developments.

While the two forms of supervision and support might have created confusion and division, this has not been the case, partly because the roles of each type of support and of the manager and practice adviser are clearly demarcated. The Joint Service's supervision policy is reproduced as an Appendix to this book.

Joint working

All the principles and philosophy of the service were based on joint working, and, to develop further, this concept required support to ensure that it really was 'joint'.

Referrals are discussed at a meeting which provides the team members with an overview of the work coming in and allows for the discussion of 'grey areas' of work. It was clear, from discussions in the earliest of these meetings, that staff were not always fully aware of the skills of other professionals and that many ideas on who does what were based on 'folk tales' and assumption rather than knowledge and experience. A useful process was a session based on 'What job I do?' – this clarified roles and identified 'grey areas' as well as establishing a basic understanding of some of the preconceived ideas that workers may have of each other's roles.

One of the principal benefits of joint working is the fact that, for many team members, shared work meant that caseloads could be increased. This allows the service to be more flexible and to offer a quicker response for people wishing to access the services available. Sharing work also meant that some people had to relinquish their sense of 'ownership' of some people's lives. For several staff this type of relationship had reduced their effectiveness and had become potentially problematic and the team managers and practice advisers were able to assess, and sometimes change, the purpose of team members' involvement with certain service users. Often staff had become stale in their approach to addressing needs, and the changes in working practice allowed them to develop a fresh perspective.

Equity and individuality

Although the service decided that the four teams should have parity, it soon became clear that four identical teams would not meet the demands which they faced locally.

It was important to allow each team autonomy to respond to the more local issues. This permitted the team managers to encourage ideas and developments amongst team members that were based on individual skills and knowledge and were additional to the core skills of each profession. Encouraging individuality in this way was also an excellent means of building ownership of the new concept of joint working in that it affirmed that the Joint Service valued individual talents. These initiatives are monitored and supervised by both the team managers and practice advisers (although an area manager or quality development officer may also be involved).

Staff must also learn to share and impart knowledge and skills rather than be perceived as the sole 'service expert' on a topic. Failure to share leads to the service losing skills when personnel leave to take up opportunities elsewhere.

Continued team-building

After the first few months, the focus of team-building needed to be changed from the staff to the service user. The themes to be addressed at this stage were:

- team objectives
- user need
- quality provision
- local networks
- project work
- continuing best practice
- forward planning.

These important issues – which had a corollary effect of building a shared vision – were developed and planned in staff teams.

Identify training needs

The continued learning needs of all staff is important and the manager, along with the practice advisers, is responsible for identifying training needs and nominating staff for internal and external courses (see also Chapter 5).

Concluding thoughts

You can lead a horse to water but you cannot make it drink.

A minority of staff will find it very difficult to come to terms with major change. Too much energy can be spent in unsuccessful attempts at persuasion and therefore it may be better, for both the service and the individual staff member, to help them consider positive career changes.

There is a danger that, in the middle of all this, the manager forgets their own needs and vulnerability. Peer and line management support is essential. The opportunities to meet with colleagues and discuss current issues and situations must be made on both a formal and informal basis. For a manager to show a level of vulnerability is acceptable so long as it is not seen as weakness which leaves the team feeling defenceless.

Figure 3. 2 shows the different stakeholders to which the team manager has to respond.

After 12 months the service attempted to move towards a more participative management style which involved staff at all levels in the future development of the service. Practical attempts to involve staff in the management process at team level have included:

- team-based working groups
- building business planning from the team level upwards
- local structures for involving senior staff in local management decisions
- delegation of some aspects of line management and work allocation to more senior staff.

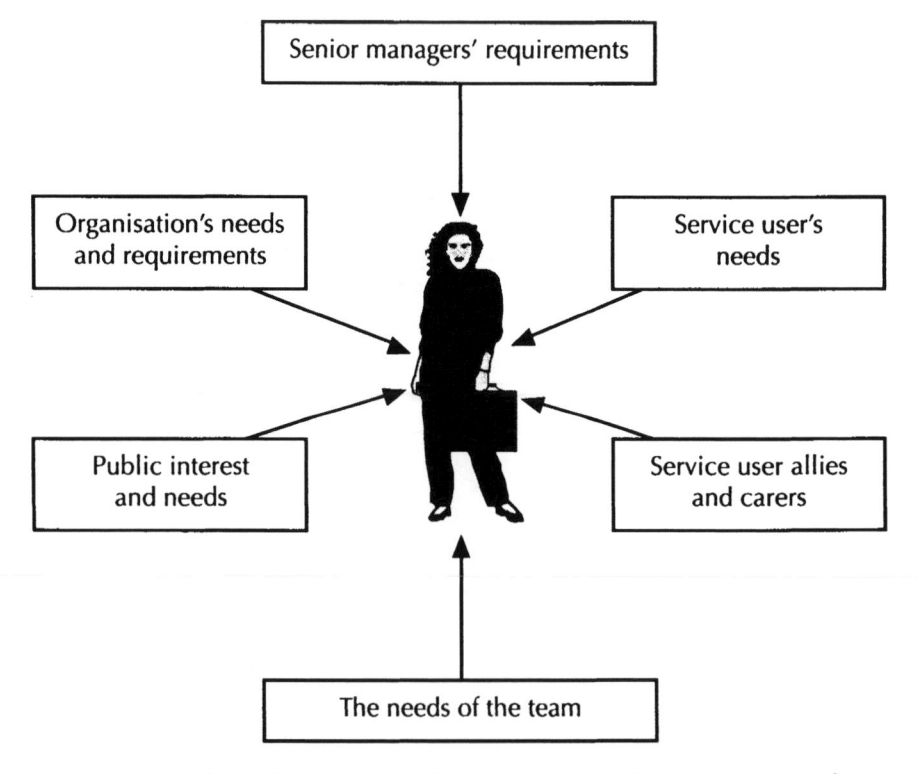

Figure 3.2   Stakeholders to whom the team manager has to be responsive

This process of participative management enables staff to recognise the effects of changing service environments in a market economy and the need for increased quality plus accountability.

The manager always has a key task to ensure that staff are positively supported in order to be able to offer the best possible service. However, it is important to remember that what works today may have to be changed tomorrow. The manager should always be prepared to learn, adapt, change and provide positive leadership towards the future.

References and resources

Adair, J. (1983), *Effective Leadership*, London: Pan Books.

Brown, S. (1990), *Community Mental Handicap Teams: Practice Papers*, London: Department of Health and University of Loughborough, Centre for Research in Social Policy.

Fisher, R., Ury, W. and Patton, B. (1991), *Getting to Yes: Negotiating an Agreement Without Giving In*, London: Random Century.

Grant, G., Humphreys, S. and McGrath, (eds) (1986), *Community Mental Handicap Teams: Theory and Practice*, Kidderminster: British Institute of Mental Handicap.
This is rather old, but covers many issues that are still relevant at the end of the 1990s.

Hastings, C., Bixby, P. and Chaudry-Lawton, R. (1986), *Superteams: A Blueprint for Organisational Success*, Glasgow: Fontana Collins.

Lawton, A. and Rose, A. (1991), *Organisation and Management in the Public Sector*, London: Pitman.

Maddux, R.B. (1988), *Team Building: An Exercise in Leadership*, London: Kogan Page.

Plant, R. (1987), *Managing Change and Making it Stick*, London: Fontana.
Includes Kurt Lewin's force field analysis.

Reder, A. (1995), *75 Best Practices for Socially Responsible Companies*, New York: Putnam.

Wilson, D.C. (1992), *A Strategy of Change: Concepts and Controversies in the Management of Change*, London: Routledge.

4 Equipping and supporting staff: residential services

Iain Larkin and Dave Ruane

Introduction

Managers' awareness of the complexities of staff support within dispersed housing networks was not simply put in place. It developed over a period of years, as the service itself developed, and continues to develop. It is, and will always be, work in progress. At one stage, staff received little, recognisable, useful support from managers, either because managers did not know what this involved, or because they did not regard it as important.

While staff supervision or job consultation is very important, it is far from being the only form of support which staff need or which managers can, or should, offer. It is essential to ensure the job to be done is understood, and that expectations are in line with both that understanding and the aims of the service.

Management cohesion

Dispersed housing networks in Manchester have been operational since the mid-1980s. The first was established in 1984, and the most recent in 1994 when Manchester's last hostel was closed.

Networks of staffed housing have replaced hospitals and hostels as the standard type of long-term support for people with learning disabilities. These networks were the culmination of a lengthy period of change and the result of a myriad smaller changes. But now they, and the philosophy behind them, are no longer the vanguard; they are a foundation stone upon which further developments in support for people with learning disabilities are being built.

Within the hostels, the staff – although generally committed to the individuals they were supporting – were encouraged to maintain a distance from them. 'Not getting emotionally involved' was a widely held tenet. The concept of 'quality of life' was largely misunderstood; individual rights, or the concept that all people belonged to their community, were still new ideas.

For some time, the networks' contact with, or effect on, the hostels was minimal. Staff from hostels and networks met only at training sessions, and the managers rarely met at all. The framework of information exchange across the wider service was not established. The benefit of the changes that occurred were hardly felt outside their immediate environment. Hostel staff, too, produced some excellent work but, because it came from a hostel, it was dismissed out of hand. They had, for example, always held 'reviews'. Hostel staff, unhappy with the format of these reviews, devised better options such as individual programme planning and person-centred planning, which were not adopted by networks for several more years, as formal planning of any sort was widely held as no longer having a legitimate function (because of misunderstandings about 'normalisation').

The sense that hostels and hostel staff were the poor relations in the whole affair and were not the sort of people you invited to dinner was very strong and did not alter until the late 1980s when a change in the senior management brought in people who understood the importance of 'the organisation' as a whole and created a structure where learning disability services were managed together.

At that time, Manchester was divided into three districts, but it was only in the very rarest circumstances that the various elements of the learning disability services came together. Different standards, policies and procedures applied to each element of the service. Within each district, the new management took the simple step of getting together representatives of each staff team from across the learning disability service on a regular monthly basis, and sharing information. It was a simple step, but probably one of the most important. Lines of communication sprang up which had never existed before, and new working relationships emerged. The developmental work undertaken in one area had a forum for evaluation and dissemination across the rest of the organisation.

It was not, of course, a straightforward process. Some professional groups could not, at first, see the value of this close relationship; network and hostels managers felt – at least initially – ignorant. Interestingly, they communicated this view to each other!

Eventually the meeting became established and practical. Its work moved away from simply getting to know each other and dealing with routine information to developing a philosophy and value-base by which the organisation could operate. One element was the framework of service accomplishments (O'Brien, 1987). Establishing a 'corporate identity' was to take several more years and go through a number of transformations, and it is still evolving now.

Having senior managers in post who shared the same perspective with each other, as well as with front-line workers, and were clearly prepared to make efforts to support network managers in propounding it amongst staff teams was a wholly new experience. It helped direct what, in hindsight, had been 'inelegant scrambling in the semi-darkness'. With that focus coming into place, managers were able to move away from a highly insular style of management to one based on shared assumptions – a stance which gave them enormous strength of purpose on the one hand, and the equipment with which they could genuinely begin to support their staff on the other. All this was continued as hostels were replaced by further dispersed networks (see Chapter 7).

The development of the Joint Service, on the lines pioneered within the south of the city, took this concept a stage further. With a functional organisational model (see Chapter 2) the main axis for development and management in the networks became the city-wide network managers' group. This group continued the programme of 'corporate development', in consultation with the rest of the organisation but more clearly targeted within the learning disability residential services. This meant that managers through the eight networks now established in the city met and devised development at one centre, not three; they coordinated developments and policy strategy, and started a process of city-wide implementation, at one centre and not three.

Standards and quality assurance

Considerable work was done by the managers and staff on developing a system of standards for internally auditing the quality of the service. This work, which is fully described in Chapter 15, also gave a shared direction to the service, with clarity about acceptable and unacceptable practices.

Expectations of the role

The critical point for staff – from the organisation's perspective – is their probationary period during which their ability to do the job is initially assessed. It is the point where staff, more than at any other time, need to be made clearly aware of what is expected of them and of the boundaries within which they must operate. However, it was a period which had been poorly used for many years. If any assessment was completed, it was ad hoc and easily challenged.

This problem was tackled by completely reviewing the process. The regrading of network support staff and the implementation of the nationally agreed benchmark criteria in 1994 gave an impetus to this change. To spread some of the load, established and experienced team members undertook the role of 'mentor' for new staff. This meant, simply, being the conduit through which the information required by new staff – on site – was passed. Responsibility for overall monitoring remained with line managers but the day-to-day knowledge of users and their histories, plus the basic running of the house, was redirected to the mentor. In addition, the probationary guidelines were rewritten, indicating in great detail all the policies and procedures which the new staff needed to read, in priority order over the 13 weeks, as well as the minimum skills they should be able to demonstrate at key points within the probationary period. These skills are linked to NVQ criteria, giving a well established baseline of competencies.

The benefits of the system are manifold:

1 Staff are more thoroughly supported during their initial 13 weeks at a minimum workload.
2 A clear decision can be made about whether their contract should be continued.
3 Staff experience an ordered induction to the job.
4 Experienced staff take on a supervision element to their role which gives them a demonstrable skill when seeking promotion.

Figure 4.1 shows the sheets used for monitoring the first four weeks of the probationary period.

Policies and procedures

To establish both standards and expectations of roles, policies had to be rewritten. Many were simply out of date; others were unclear and poorly put together. Some necessary policies did not exist. At one time, there had been a 'manual of guidance' for managers, detailing the current policies within social services, but it had not operated since 1985 and no efforts were being made to revive it. The inevitable result was that few policies were being appropriately held to and people's understanding of them was frequently wrong.

Week 1–4

> Name of Probationer: ....
> Date of Commencement:...
> Name of Mentor: ....
> Name of ANM: ....

How many work days have been missed over this period because of

sickness [ ] any other reason [ ]

Have there been any incidents of lateness

yes [ ] (how many [ ])   no [ ]

Information Exchanged

Date completed   Signed

Read PRS* Files

Read tenant profiles/histories

Read handover files

Layout of house/
where things are

* Personal Record System.   *cont'd*

Figure 4.1 Sample sheets for monitoring probationary staff induction

Tenant occupation:
visit to college etc.

Policies and Procedures

NSW Job Description

Finance policy/procedure

Medication policy

Hepatitis B inoculation

Smoking policy

Alcohol policy

Annual leave

Fire procedure

Figure 4.1   concluded

The management group began to collate and rewrite policies. It was an extensive business, but the exercise was beneficial in that managers became familiar with them and, through discussion, were interpreting them similarly. As a consequence of this, much time was spent cascading the information through to the staff teams and checking, via written confirmation, that each of them had received and read them.

Best practice

Policies written in their traditional format can be dry and dull. This can be resolved in two ways – by clearly defining the 'dos and don'ts' of the particular issue, within the policy, and also by producing working documents such as the *The Best Practice Guide*. This document was initially composed by the staff themselves and comprised a series of pithy statements of good and bad practice. However, over time, it has become a tool for inducting new staff – a way of introducing policies to new staff without boring them to distraction.

Discipline

Having undertaken the task of redrafting policies, we were obliged to enforce them. Typically, managers within local authorities were poor at discipline. They were themselves untrained. They had little or no experience in how to use the disciplinary codes and little or no support in using it. Furthermore, while services were so disparate, there was a sense that, if a member of staff was taken to task, it reflected very badly on the manager him or herself and that a breach of discipline 'proved' in some way that he or she could not cope. Consequently, some very serious breaches of discipline went unchallenged by anything more than a 'word in the ear'. This gave the more unscrupulous staff members a *carte blanche* and resulted, for many years, in a situation where bad staff were effectively protected by the system. Good staff became demoralised and afraid to 'blow the whistle' in case they were somehow implicated or left to suffer the consequences.

Learning to enforce an organisation's policies was not easy; managers still had to risk losing disciplinary actions. However, the fact that the managers themselves had written many of the policies – so there was a sense of real ownership of the issue – and that, because of the closer union between the networks as a whole, managers had a better support network made it considerably easier. The sense of belonging to a larger team – of having obligations not just to service users and other staff, but to the wider organisation – was very effective in encouraging managers to take that first step in disciplining errant staff. This process:

- reinforced policies and underlined the need to ensure that managers took the time and energy to make all staff aware of policies
- improved morale for many staff
- encouraged staff to deal with bad practice, either by reporting it – knowing that they would be supported in resolving it – or directly by bringing poor staff into line with the immediate team's approach (see below)
- re-emphasised the high standards of the service with each disciplinary action taken.

Building teams

Like many other aspects of managing, the importance of the 'team' is something which becomes understood over time. In hostels the team existed largely in name only; they were a collection of people who shared a rota pattern or worked with the same group of people. Once networks became the principal form of support, the importance of teamwork began to be more keenly realised, as staff had to deal with the very real stresses and strains of working in isolation from each other. Our understanding of its real importance has now grown to a point where we have begun to actively draw on the pool of staff in order to try and create more complementary and effective teams.

Because of the comparatively high turnover of staff in residential services, work with service users became circular in nature. For example, one group of staff might undertake skill development with a user and then be transferred or disbanded. The subsequent team would identify the same skill deficiencies and begin the same process, although perhaps in a different way. Users might endure generations of staff tinkering, moving on and being tinkered with again by someone else to little effect.

We instigated a system of maintaining a core group of staff, effectively agreeing with those staff, locally, that they would not be moved from that team for a given period of anything up to two years (unless, of course, a major issue arose which could not be resolved otherwise). This group of people then took responsibility for actively progressing work with users.

Newer staff were brought into that team, but were not offered 'permanency' until it was clear that they had settled. As new people joined the core it allowed existing staff to be released, if they wanted or needed to move on. In this way the team became more than the sum of its members; it became a culture which worked for the service users.

This strategy cannot always work. However, it was backed up through the use of active team-building methods which varied from half-day brainstorming sessions to simple exercises at the beginning of each fortnightly team meeting. Line managers found that those teams which were well balanced very largely 'managed' themselves; the teams' pride in their work was such that the rules of conduct for individual members were quite strict and poor work was dealt with promptly by colleagues.

This also partly resolved a considerable problem of line managers managing effectively from a distance. Teamwork can take on some of this role, although it would be damaging to allow it to go too far.

The teams' communication skills developed too. Communication is based on mutual understanding, not just of language, but of the more idiosyncratic nuances of speech and behaviour. The closer the ties within the group, the greater was the quality of their communication. The standard of recording improved, as did the effectiveness of the team meetings.

Project work

The wider team facilitated development although, in this instance, the benefits we discovered were accidental.

The Joint Service has established a reputation for getting things done. After a slow start, where most people – still traumatised by successive years of 'restructuring' – were inclined to pessimism, various projects were implemented.

Our first problem was the reduction, in the city, of available day care for people we supported. In an effort to combat the situation, two 'drop-ins' were set up in the south of the city. One was run for people with very significant disabilities, where the input was organised and specific. The second was an open session, with a wide variety of activities, but with no particular onus to undertake anything – a social affair. Both proved highly successful and spawned a series of related projects. The key projects were the Telesafe Video Project (see Chapter 13) and the Sessional Worker Project. The Sessional Worker Project was based on an idea developed by the resettlement programme in Manchester. The coordinating staff – who are network staff – undertook to match volunteers (who are paid a fee for their time by the user) to people with a learning disability on the basis of a shared interest. They implemented a full vetting procedure, and offered basic training to volunteers new into this area. The scheme supported people who lived in networks and in the local community and has proved to be both successful and valuable to the people who use it.

However, the success of projects such as these lies as much in their ripple effects as in their main intent. The ripple effects come through the staff team as a whole. Project work invariably involves substantial effort. Projects have been successful because they offer individual staff a release from their routine work and a sense of kudos and pride in their completion. Staff have put enormous energy into some projects and, overall, the Joint Service has created a variety of additional resources available to learning-disabled people – for example, an allotment group, an art group, community safety videos and 'chance to meet' discos.

Some of the projects undertaken fail, but those that do work spark off a series of other projects in which staff from different networks or different teams get together and devise simple but imaginative responses to a need.

We have enhanced this practice now, so that when a more formal project is proposed, such as a suggested area for training or a potential planning strategy for users, we habitually advertise throughout the Joint Service for people who have an interest in developing the idea. This brings in people who are genuinely interested and continues the process of widening the working team from one house or one network to the full service.

Management changes

The reorganisation of the service involved one key change in 1994 which had largely unexpected outcomes for the development of the staff teams. This was the move from senior residential social workers (RSWs) to assistant network managers (ANMs).

Senior RSWs were hands-on managers; they worked within the teams, on rota and monitored the work directly. The problem was that, in times of staff shortage, seniors might spend most of their time working in the houses and have insufficient time to be effective managers. Creating the ANMs, who were more clearly part of the management team, involved reducing the number of these managers by nearly half (and increasing the number of direct support staff with the money saved) and making each ANM responsible for two to three staff teams.

An initial concern was how teams would function without direct hands-on support. We still maintained a directive approach to staff. However, after an initial settling-in period, staff became more self-reliant, taking decisions which would previously have been left until a senior arrived. They initiated work, where previously they may have waited to be directed. They organised rota changes, where previously they would have left it for the senior.

This was counterbalanced by the ANM's own skill growth. The standard of management skill within the seniors was very variable; they operated with continual reference to the network manager. However, the extra tasks allocated to the ANM meant that this system could not continue, and ANMs quickly had to develop distance management skills – plan, communicate and prioritise more effectively. They needed to delegate and be more focused in their approach, and this was how they responded.

The most problematic area was monitoring standards. ANMs were concerned that they would be unable to ensure that work practices would not deteriorate. Yet staff, given the responsibility, did demonstrate their commitment to the people they were supporting.

Where breaches of discipline did occur, ANMs responded differently, too. The greater distance between manager and team naturally lead to two things – an awareness that policies and procedures needed to be clearly passed on and kept to, and a firmer response to instances where procedures were required.

Previously, the typical response to a disciplinary issue was to 'talk it through' with the staff member and, because seniors and their staff team worked so closely together, this very frequently meant that some serious issues were brushed under the carpet. Now, because a distance had been established, ANMs were able to deal with them more appropriately.

In turn, this meant that other staff, who had felt undermined by the non-resolution of poor practice, understood that they would receive support and were more inclined to actively raise issues themselves in the future.

Formal supports

Job consultation, or supervision, as it was formerly known, has been one of two formal support settings for staff in the Joint Service for several years. It pre-dates the service by some considerable time, but its previous poor implementation left many staff deeply cynical of its value.

In order to re-establish it, we undertook a lengthy consultation exercise amongst both staff and managers, backed by the development of a clear policy document which more tightly bounded the responsibilities of the line manager and the realm of the discussions which should take place.

The function of the job consultation is threefold – advice, support and management – but it is based upon a two-way discussion and not simply a 'grilling' by a manager. We impressed upon staff that the sessions would deal with their agendas, as well as management agendas, but in either case outcomes must be expected. For the process to be continuous, it was not simply a matter of holding regular job consultations it also required routinely reviewing previous discussions at the start of the next session. A written job consultation record became, essentially, a contract between the two parties, and both the staff member's and the manager's progress needed to be checked. The original policy was amended over time by including standing agenda items. The purpose of this was not to exclude any particular discussion, but rather to ensure that specific topics were regularly discussed. These were:

- Previous minutes
- Training: skill development
- New policies
- Sickness record
- Information briefing (various meetings).

The issue of 'confidentiality' was also raised routinely, so that the groundrules for the session were clear.

Self-assessment has also been introduced into job consultation. This is a simple format whereby staff members and their line managers complete the same assessment form. It looks at the range of skills and aptitudes relating to the support worker role. Where differences in rating appear, an agenda item for discussion is found. Low scores indicate a skill deficit, or training need; high scores indicate an achieved competency. Although staff and managers are aware that it is an informal system designed purely to establish a basis for future work, it has proven very useful in identifying differences in perceptions of individual staff skills.

Team meetings have a similar function to job consultations; they enable group planning and discussion sessions, where issues can be tackled on an even footing. The success of the these meetings is largely dependent on the skill of the manager running the session. It is important, for example, to ensure that those topics with which everyone is involved – the lives of the tenants – remain at the top.

Discussing key issues each session enables them to be resolved quickly. Other business items, properly prioritised and time-limited, should ensure that the majority of business is dealt with on time, and to everyone's satisfaction.

We have discovered – again, following the example of one particular manager – that beginning each session with a brief team-building exercise does two things. It continues the process of team bonding, which remains a critical factor in service delivery as expectations of teams increases, and it draws a very clear line between previous discussions and the start of the session. It is easier to manage any (temporary) ill-feeling between staff by putting the meeting into its own context.

Informal support: management by walking about

Managers often seem to view support as something you do to people – something separate from their other responsibilities – yet to see it in such a light is to miss an opportunity.

Managers, by using such phrases as 'My door is always open' possibly do greater damage to the effectiveness of an individual member of staff or staff team than by almost any other means, as it sets up an immediate barrier. The message it sends is that staff must seek out managers, and it does nothing to diminish the perceived barrier between management and staff.

Accessibility is not just a matter of being available: it is being seen to be available. Many problems are solved more easily by meeting staff in casual settings than in formal settings. Apart from the routine monitoring exercise, when managers are obliged to visit houses to complete network inspections or similar, they must make it an habitual practice to 'drop in' without invitation to see how things are going. This helps to ensure that staff remain conscious of their practice and that managers have an up-to-date account of events within the house. It clearly demonstrates managers' willingness to make the effort to go to the staff, rather than the staff always having to come and find them. Staff do make use of this time to deal with minor issues such as complaints and the like, which may otherwise remain unresolved and problematic. And, for a great many staff, it is the minor irritants which cause greatest grief.

A final point for managers to consider is their own role in maintaining staff morale. Managers need to have the pressure under which they work recognised and to receive support in overcoming these periods as much as any other member of staff. The relationship many managers have with their staff is such that much of the support they need can be gained from this group. Whilst this is informal it is extremely valuable. But this is a specific relationship which is built up, over time, amongst people who have usually worked as direct colleagues; it is not automatic.

Conclusion

This chapter has described the changes that took place over a period of three or four years. They were required as a result of a substantial change in the mode of service delivery – from 24-person hostels to supported living in ordinary houses.

It is important to recognise the scale of these changes and the consequent impact on both the people receiving these services and those delivering them.

Hostels	Supported Living
• A single large building-based service.	• A dispersed service provided in people's homes
• A service provided by low-paid, often manually graded staff with a clear demarcation of roles – for example, handyman/driver, cooks, secretaries	• Support staff paid on Administrative Professional and Technical grade (APTG) who are responsible for all the tasks involved in enabling a person to live in the community.
• Residents comprising mainly people with moderate to severe disability.	• User group increasingly including people with severe to profound and multiple disability
• Low expectation of involvement in the community. People were largely invisible behind the front door of the hostel. Family assumed that they were going into a 'home for life'.	• High expectation of taking a full part in their community. People are highly visible to neighbours, family and trades-people. There is an expectation that people will develop their skills and opportunities.
• Staff and managers working within a narrow residential, 'social' care service.	• Staff and managers are part of a wider context of service provision which includes health and social care.
• Quality control more or less limited to annual inspections.	• A matrix of checks and balances in place to ensure that standards are established and monitored and that quality is built into everyday operations.

References

O'Brien, J. (1987), 'A guide to personal futures planning', in G. T. Bellamy and B. Wilcox (eds), *The Activities Catalogue: A Community Programming Guide for Youths and Adults with Severe Learning Disabilities*, Baltimore: Brookes-Cole.

5 Joint training

Pauline John

Introduction

With the introduction of increased competition and the purchaser–provider split, it is vital to recognise the importance of training in developing and maintaining a high-quality service. Organisations sometimes view training as a short-term gain or 'quick fix' solution to complex issues. When budgets become tight, training can be the first item to 'fall off the end'. Certainly it is often a 'Cinderella' in the wider organisational context.

However, investment in training and developing the workforce is a long-term strategy that, over time, ensures a higher quality of care and better motivated staff. Training significantly contributes to a well managed service, especially in terms of good practice and policy development.

Key issues: policy and provision

Over the past decade there has been a considerable shift in how services are delivered. There are greater expectations of services both in terms of standards and outcomes. The contract culture of service provision has become tighter and the issue of quality is higher on the agenda.

Public services now often follow the pattern of private industries in promoting their services by achieving nationally agreed measures and standards of good quality – for example, Investors in People, Charter Marks and training awards. Griffiths (1991) drew close comparisons between public and private sector:

> The clear similarities between NHS management and business management are much more important. In many organisations in the private sector, profit does not immediately impinge on large numbers of managers below board level. They are concerned with levels of service, quality of produce, monitoring and rewarding staff, research and development, and the long term viability of the undertaking. (Griffiths, 1991)

For better or worse, there has been a change in focus for public service organisations into that of the competitive market. When reviewing the literature about nationally agreed frameworks such as National Vocational Qualifications (NVQs) or Investors in People, the language of business, management and competitive markets is appropriated into the world of training and development:

> Public sector organisations which are to succeed, thrive and maintain influence in a competitive climate are those which have a keen understanding of their client's needs, a sense of values which underpin their business and a management and staff whose skills are overt, highly developed and capable of meeting a complex range of ever changing tasks. Successful care organisations will be those who place the development of competence at the heart of the workforce policies. (NVQ Criteria & Guidance, 1996)

The notion of competence is central to the NVQ framework. Within companies, NVQs are being encouraged on the basis that they can improve business performance by bringing a more focused attitude to training to meet business objectives.

The Investors in People standard was launched at the CBI conference in 1990. One of the key issues on which Investors in People focuses is how organisations evaluate the benefits of training:

> The Investors In People approach treats the process of 'people developments' in the same way as any other major business investment. It focuses people's activity and their training and development on the achievement of business goals and targets. It ensures that the investment in training and development provides 'value for money'. (Investors In People (Scotland) Evaluation of Training – *Guidance for Managers*)

To achieve any of these awards, training must remain high on the organisation's priorities.

It is generally recognised that joint working between organisations in the provision of services is desirable (see Chapter 1). To ensure that good joint working exists between staff from different backgrounds and perspectives, a shared understanding of roles and responsibilities is important. Much of that can be achieved through joint training initiatives.

Experience in Manchester: establishing a joint training approach

The establishment of the Joint Service in April 1994 allowed for greater flexibility and richness in the provision of training across the service. Having a single management structure enabled the management team to set its priorities for the service, which ensure that both health and social services staff were working to shared aims and objectives. Recognising the value of training within a large service, the management team made training a priority for the service and give it a high profile on the organisational agenda.

Before the establishment of the Joint Service in April 1994, there were different mechanisms for the provision of training across the city. South Manchester already had a joint model of provision which recognised the importance of training. It had set up a training action group (TAG) which consisted of a variety of interested health and social services staff, and was chaired by a member of the management team. This group had an oversight of all training within the service. This originally consisted of generic training, which came from the local social services department training base, and a small budget from the Health Authority, used to fund health staff on more specific training.

There had been little training for front-line staff on issues that affected their day-to-day practice. Very few courses had been jointly run. Budgetary issues were a constraint, with little money to pay for courses that were often very expensive.

The group had a vision of how training might be organised and developed within the service. Their main strengths were enthusiasm and a genuine commitment to improving service provision, by delivering appropriate training to the workforce.

The South Manchester TAG devised a model of organising training which capitalised on the specialist skills and knowledge of those staff within the service. In conjunction with line managers, a number of training needs were identified for front-line staff to enable them to perform their job effectively.

The TAG commissioned a number of core courses, including a Basic Induction for all new staff, Personal and Intimate Care and Epilepsy (many service users have epilepsy, and many staff had little knowledge of the condition). A course on Epilepsy was designed by two community nurses and the Personal and Intimate Care course was designed and delivered by one of the physiotherapists. These courses then began to run on a rolling programme across the south of the city.

At that stage, it was important to achieve small successes which could act as a foundation for future training initiatives. The emphasis was on quality rather than quantity. It was also important to establish a culture where training was high on the agenda. This would have been difficult to achieve if the staff attending the training did not feel it to be appropriate or of value. The TAG wanted to have training which staff felt was worth attending, and that was not viewed in any way as being second-rate.

The model had also used by both the Central and North districts of the city with slightly differing emphasis and mixed success. When the city-wide service was established in April 1994, a city-wide training action group was created. The membership, as before, reflected the broad range of roles and services across the city. The city-wide group adopted the same approach as that used in South Manchester. The same process of creating small successes commenced.

Benefits of joint training

The Joint Service has been able to extend the range of courses available to front-line staff. As both health and social care professionals are managed by the service, they are able to provide training in their specific areas of expertise to basic grade workers. Examples of this include:

- the Role of The Appropriate Adult course, which was designed and is delivered by two care managers
- training in the very specialist area of Alternative and Augmented Communication, delivered by speech and language therapists.

Because these staff are part of the service, the management team is able to build the training role into their defined workload.

Being part of a larger community health trust also provides enormous benefits in terms of access to other specialist professional staff. Two good examples of this are training that is run by the dietetics department, on food and nutrition, and the dental department on oral health. These specialist health professionals design and deliver these courses in conjunction with the Joint Service so that they are relevant to the needs of people with learning disabilities.

All staff, from senior managers through to basic grade staff, share the same understanding of how training is coordinated and organised throughout the service. The TAG, drawing on a cross-section of staff and managers, has become an established arm of the organisation.

The city-wide TAG brochure is published on a six-monthly basis and contains details of all the training that is available for that period. Details of course aims and objectives, the target group of staff, course trainers and specific guidance for managers is contained within the brochure. It also outlines the mission statement of the group and the group objectives:

> The Training Action Group will ensure that there is a rolling programme of high quality training available to all staff within learning disability services. All training will be developed and planned in line with the current and predicted tasks faced by the service. Every person employed by the Joint Service is a valued and skilled part of a team. The overall aim of the training group is to further develop and expand that individually based skill, and so enhance the service. (TAG brochure, 1996)

It is interesting to note that the model used in learning disability services in Manchester is viewed as a system of promoting good practice in the organisation and management of training in any given service. It is being replicated within the social services department's purchaser and provider divisions.

Why did the TAG work?

There were a number of factors which contributed to the overall success of the TAG as a fully functional group which could demonstrate its achievements over a sustained period. One of the principal factors was having a committed senior manager within the organisation leading the group. Personal interest, coupled with the seniority of the position, meant that, as chair of the group, there was a real ability to 'make things happen' and negotiate at a senior level.

As part of the overall management style within the service, objectives are set on a six-monthly basis. The senior manager with responsibility for training in the organisation has a clear objective to produce a six-monthly training schedule for the service. This is viewed as a significant part of the manager's workload and is accommodated within the Joint Service management group.

Second, the overall composition of the group is important in terms of the group's success. The group is representative of the various roles within the organisation and includes people with differing levels of responsibility. There is a requirement that members of the group are active participants. They are required to represent the interests of a specific group of staff and to provide feedback to that group. They are also required to contribute to the overall aim of the group by taking on some additional work. This may be in the form of providing some direct training, coordinating a group which is developing a training course, making external contacts, or some other organisational task connected to training, but not necessarily within the context of their professional role within the service.

The group membership has comprised motivated staff and managers who have a personal interest and commitment to training, take their role within the group seriously and enjoy the benefits that being a participant bring. With such an active membership, members who do not actively participate are easily identified; these people are then offered the opportunity to either improve or leave the group.

The other key member of the group is the the quality development officer who is able to bring a technical dimension to the workings of the group, up-to-date information about new developments in training and ideas on how to demonstrate good-quality outcomes in training as part of ongoing evaluation and improvements.

Embedding training into the organisational culture

It is worth emphasising the importance of training within an organisation and promoting training as a significant part of a workforce's workload. It was therefore important to ensure that the TAG had a high profile within the service, which was understood by staff at all levels. This was done in a number of ways:

1   Training is a standard agenda item at the monthly Joint Service management meeting. It is expected that the chair of the TAG will ensure, through this standing agenda item, that all the other senior managers within the service are fully informed and updated, in terms of what is going on, any potential problems, conflicts or agreements, and about future directions and developments.
2   The chair of the TAG, through the Joint Service management group, also ensures that specific news items about training are regularly briefed to staff.
3   Training is also given a high profile through the network monitoring system. Network managers must make regular returns which show how many staff received what training over the previous month. This specifically sets out an expectation that network staff will receive regular training, and this is audited.

Organisation of training in the Joint Service

Training is divided into four main categories:

1   Underpinning Knowledge

2 Supporting Learning Disability Needs
3 Supporting Additional Health Needs
4 Staff and Management Responsibilities.

Examples from each section are as follows:

1 Underpinning Knowledge:

 – Induction
 – Service Philosophy.

2 Supporting Learning Disability Needs:

 – Alternative and Augmentative Language Communication Workshop
 – Risk Taking.

3 Supporting Additional Health Needs:

 – Epilepsy Levels 1 and 2
 – Mental Health & Learning Disabilities Levels 1 and 2
 – First Aid: The First Few Minutes.

4 Staff and Management Responsibilities:

 – Train the Trainers
 – Chairing Meetings.

An example of the First Aid training can be seen in Figure 5.1.

As training has developed through the service and TAG process it has become more sophisticated. The TAG is currently looking at linking training to job descriptions by identifying core competencies for all levels of staff within the organisation. Work has now been completed for domiciliary care staff and network support workers where five core competencies were agreed as the basic core elements required. An audit was conducted across the service to establish how many staff had already completed the core training, so that sufficient core training could be included in the forthcoming training schedules.

The results of the audit are reported in Table 5.1.

In line with the notion of core competencies, the TAG, through its strong links with Manchester social services training section, has commenced work on linking its training to competencies identified as part of the NVQ system. By endeavouring to tailor in-house courses to the needs of NVQ it ensures that attendance on TAG courses can contribute to the evidence-gathering necessary for competence-based training. To date, this has been achieved on the following courses: Personal and Intimate Care; First Aid –

First Aid

Aims:

To provide the participants with sufficient knowledge and confidence in the initial assistance and treatment of a person who has had an accident or injury before the arrival of an ambulance, doctor or other qualified personnel.

Objectives:
1. Participants will understand the basic principles of breathing and circulation.
2. Participants will understand the basic principles of the recovery position.
3. Participants will be aware of basic principles of resuscitation and the steps that should be taken on the discovery of a collapsed person.
4. Participants will have a practical knowledge of how to deal with the following:

Wounds and bleeding;
Burns and scalds;
Choking;
Basic bandaging techniques;
Household accidents.

Figure 5.1   Example of a First Aid training course

Table 5.1   Results of the core training audit

	Induction	Moving & Handling	Food Hygiene	Personal & Intimate Care	First Aid
	%	%	%	%	%
Network support workers	69	66	65	49	31
Waking night staff	53	61	–	26	3
Domiciliary carers	51	88	84	70	59

The First Few Minutes; Risk Taking; Epilepsy; Abuse of Vulnerable Adults. Work is under way on a range of other courses.

Budgetary issues

In times of tight budgetary control, training has to be approached as creatively as possible. Managers are required to organise and manage rotas as effectively as possible if staff are to be released for training.

In turn, the TAG has addressed the issue by implementing a variety of different training methods, focusing on cost-effectiveness. This is demonstrated in the following examples:

- Key training was condensed from a full day to a four-hour session which can be put on locally at convenient times – for example, 12–4 pm.
- The Joint Service is currently exploring the possibility of developing video-based training materials for certain courses, which staff could either view during team meetings or take home. The first two will be a refresher for Manual Handling and Personal and Intimate Care.
- In the audit of core training it was identified that night support workers and network support workers had received very little core training in First Aid – The First Few Minutes course. Releasing night staff to be trained during the day and then covering their shifts is very costly, so an alternative way of addressing this need had to be found. The two lead trainers are community nurses based in one of the community teams. It was agreed that for a period of one week they would work nights and would deliver a revised training course on a one-to-one basis at specified sites. A follow-up evaluation will assess how effective this training has been. It is assumed that one-to-one training will be as, or more, effective than receiving training in a large group. Revising the work patterns of community nurses is a more cost-effective method of delivering training than releasing night staff and covering their shifts.

Income generation

When the TAG was initially established, it had no allocated resources. The principle of using employed staff to be lead trainers in certain areas of specification was its only resource. As the group has become more established and sophisticated it has been able to generate a certain amount of income.

The Joint Service is the largest statutory provider organisation in Manchester. It is therefore able to offer training to other smaller independent providers in the city, as well as the remaining social services direct provision. The TAG's core business aim is to provide good-quality training for its own staff group (which exceeds 600 staff). However, places are sold on courses to other providers and, where possible, specific sessions are tailored to the independent sector where there are sufficient numbers. Prices are usually based on a per person per course basis. The income generated is then reinvested in training, by either funding staff to do additional training that is not available in-house, or by buying in training that is specialist in nature. The benefit for the independent providers is that they receive good-quality training at considerably reduced rates.

Evaluation

Evaluation of training has always been a key issue for services. Is the organisation's investment in training ensuring that it meets its objectives? Are the desired outcomes of training met? Has practice changed and improved as a result of training? To answer these questions some method of evaluation needs to be employed. Some methodologies are complex and time-consuming; some are quite quick and easy. The organisation needs to make decisions on which to use and which methods will be most useful.

The TAG has targeted evaluation on specific courses to ensure that the training:

- meets course objectives
- changes practice/makes improvements to practice
- enables learning to be retained.

At the end of each course an evaluation or 'instant reaction sheet' is completed. This asks general questions about quality of tutor, course content, useful/least useful sessions, and whether there was anything missing from the course. Although this method has been dismissed by many as being nothing more than 'happy sheets', they have given a gauge of how participants have felt after attending the course. However, they are clearly unable to measure effectiveness in the workplace.

To address the issue of effectiveness the quality development officer, in conjunction with the TAG, identified a series of key courses in which outcomes would be more closely examined. Over time, a number of methods were used.

- **Method one**. A questionnaire was sent to both the course participant and the relevant line manager approximately three months after course attendance. The questionnaire asked both the participant and manager if there had been any pre-course discussion regarding the training, and any post-course follow-up. It also asked whether practice had changed and to give examples of this.

- **Method two.** Course participants and managers were interviewed by the quality development officer approximately three months after course attendance. Similar questions were asked as in method one.

Both methods offered the organisation useful information, but the general conclusions were as follows:

- Interviews gleaned the most information regarding the quality and content of the course, and how practice may or may not have changed. On the other hand, they were time-consuming to arrange.
- Course participants who had input from their managers both before and after the course were more likely to have directly applied the course to their work, or felt it had changed the lives of the service users they had worked with.

As a result of this first evaluation of three TAG courses, a further three were identified for evaluation.

Some changes were made to the questions that were asked. More emphasis was given to change in practice and knowledge retention. To establish this, the course tutor was asked to contribute to the formulation of the questionnaire. Specific questions were tabled to test the knowledge and practice of the staff member after attending the course.

Examples are as follows:

- **Manual Handling training.** In two different scenarios staff were asked what action they would take when faced with a specific situation. The questions were designed to find out whether people would attempt to manage the situation on their own (this was the incorrect answer), or know to refer to a physiotherapist, either directly or through a manager (correct answer).
- **Epilepsy Level One training.** Staff were asked how they would deal with a specific epileptic episode while out at the park. They were asked what steps they would take both immediately and after the seizure had finished.
- **Induction.** Three scenarios were given to find out if participants were clear as to who they would expect to carry out work with specific service users. This was mainly to test the understanding of roles within the community team.

The service has found these evaluations to be beneficial in the following ways:

- They check that core objectives are being met.
- They ensure that practice reflects training – that is, its quality and impact on service users' lives are improved.
- They ensure that participants have retained key information in relation to the subject.
- They ensure the link between management and staff in the identification of training and in pre- and post-training discussion.

Conclusion

This chapter has described the place of training within the work of the Joint Service. Training is a major investment and has a critical impact on the quality and retention of staff. If public sector providers are to compete on a "best value" basis with independent sector providers, they need highly skilled and motivated staff. The Joint Service capitalises on the talents within its own staff group and accesses the training opportunities of both the social services department and the Trust.

The TAG has been effective in providing a large amount of training over a wide range of subjects. Led by a senior manager and comprising staff from a range of professions and working situations, it has established a key place within the organisation. Each course is quality controlled and evaluated over time. The Joint Service audits regularly whether the training programme is meeting staff needs and attempts to rectify shortfalls in provision. The TAG has developed a number of imaginative responses to providing training within tight budgetary constraints.

As a large statutory provider, the Joint Service, has a responsibility to offer training opportunities to smaller independent providers and to help them set standards and procedures of good practice.

References

Griffiths, Sir R. (1991), cited in J.R.N. Bullivant (ed) (1994), *Benchmarking for Continuous Improvement in the Public Sector*, Harlow: Longman Information and Reference.

Investors in People (1994), cited in J.R.N. Bullivant (ed), *Benchmarking for Continuous Improvement in the Public Sector*, Harlow: Longman Information and Reference.

NVQ Criteria & Guidance (1996), *Letter to Directors of Social Services*, Association of County Councils, Local Government Management Board, Council for Education and Training in Social Work and Association of Directors of Social Services.

6 Producing and implementing effective policies

Pauline John and Mark Burton

Introduction

In Chapter 2 we distinguished between simple control, technical control, professional control and bureaucratic control. In the case of bureaucratic control, work tasks and procedures are formalised, made predictable and standardised. Formal policies are one way of achieving this formalisation. However, the creation of policies can also serve some more developmental functions. We can regard policies as tools that:

1 identify the responsibilities of both staff and the organisation
2 provide guidance to staff
3 clarify the aims of the organisation and the means by which it reaches them.

It is common to regard policies as 'boring but necessary', but their production can be a creative process that allows opportunities for the building of a consensus on required, desirable, as well as unacceptable, actions.

Key issues

Policies and procedures

It is useful to distinguish between policies and procedures. Policies may contain procedures, but tend to have a wider scope and may be less prescriptive than procedures.

Level, scope and specificity

Policies may operate at different levels of the organisation and, indeed, of the service system. In the north-west, a regional health authority policy ('The Model District Service'), which was also endorsed by other organisations, exerted considerable influence on learning disability services throughout Lancashire and Greater Manchester. Some policies are the policies of the organisation as a whole, such as an NHS trust, a social services department, or a national voluntary organisation. Others may be the policy of one division of an organisation. At the other extreme, a policy may be something that one service element – for example, a community team or a day service – works to.

Clarity

Policies must be clear enough to give guidance that can be interpreted unambiguously. It can take several attempts to get this right: the process of consultation will help with this.

Ownership

Policies which do not have the assent of those who will be affected by them will be difficult to operate. The building of ownership is important throughout the development and implementation of policies. It can help to involve the key stakeholders in their production and to consult widely, perhaps with more limited consultations on early drafts.

Implementation and review

As Labour Party activists discovered in the 1980s, there is more to the promotion of change than the agreement of policies! Staff must be briefed and possibly trained in them; there may also be a need for supporting documentation and for key people to take on new responsibilities. Policies generally require some kind of monitoring and periodically require review and modification as circumstances change and experience suggests improvements. For this reason, the production of policies should not be embarked on lightly – a great deal of work may be required, so an effective organisation will keep policies to the minimum required for efficient, safe and effective functioning.

Practical guidance

The following guide outlines the steps involved in policy production, with key issues to consider at each step.

So you think you need a policy?

Identify the need that the policy is intended to meet, for example:

- guidance to staff in a difficult area
- rights of service users
- clarification of roles and responsibilities

What would be the scope of the policy?

This means identifying the appropriate section of the service to which the policy applies, for example:

- one unit or team – for example, guidance on the use of a particular resource or feature of the setting, such as the reception area, or piloting of a new approach, such as a crisis intervention facility
- one division – for example, day services
- the whole organisation
- the local service system – for example, guidance on defining eligibility for service, procedures for dealing with allegations of abuse.

Who else thinks you need a policy?

Does the appropriate management level also see the need for a policy? If not, and you still think it will be useful, is it worth considering piloting the policy at a local level? Local policies are often adopted by organisations. Will this management level ratify the policy, and do they understand its implications?

Is there a person or group with lead responsibility for policy development?

Such a person or group is useful to prevent proliferation of incompatible policies. If they exist it will also be important to involve them, seek advice or get permission to proceed. Is that person or group able to manage the workload effectively, negotiate at senior level, secure agreements of the key players? Is there a clear mandate and remit?

Is there access to administrative support?

This is important for arranging meetings, and managing the paperwork involved.

How will the policy be written?

It is worth considering how to build in the involvement of others. Methods that have worked well include the following:

- **An initial workshop or conference**. This surfaces and explores the issues and possible solutions.
- **A collective writing session**. One useful approach is to draw up a list of issues to be covered with each group member taking one issue and writing a rough draft of that section of the policy. As they finish, they pass their piece on to someone else, who suggests amendments and makes constructive comments; the pieces of paper can be passed on several times to gather a wide range of commentary and amendment. This results in a great deal of quickly produced material which can then be edited into a first draft of the policy.
- **Review**. One person writes a review of the particular topic, which is then discussed before writing the policy. This works well for the more technical areas.

Consultation

Once a first draft has been prepared, the consultation process can begin. It may be worth doing a limited consultation in the first place, to identify any obvious mistakes and issues that would adversely affect a wider consultation. Once a reasonably mature draft has been made, then a wider consultation might be carried out.

Who do you need to consult with? Consider the following to decide.

1   What is the purpose of the policy?
2   Who is involved?
3   Who will be affected?
4   Whose agreement would be necessary or desirable?

Possible groups to consult include:

- other statutory and independent providers
- personnel departments

- the health authority
- registration and inspection departments
- service users and their organisations
- families of service users
- advocates
- carers
- education providers
- professional groups and advisers
- other agencies (housing, police, probation)
- legal advisers
- contract managers.

It is worth marking each draft with its edition number (for example, 'draft 1', 'final draft for agreement') and date. For a wide consultation it is worth numbering each copy and asking for it to be returned with annotations. This prevents confusion about the status of the different versions of a policy that might end up in circulation and reinforces the consultative nature of the process (the policy is only a draft until the consultation is over).

Decide when to stop consulting, and how you will resolve differences of opinion.

Ratification

The policy will need ratifying by the management group, board or committee with responsibility for the services to which it applies. It is difficult to be prescriptive about this, but two examples from our own service may help.

1 *Responding to Violence and Aggression* (including policy on the use of physical intervention). There was wide consultation with all those on the above list. Ratification was provided by both the trust board and by the Social Services Committee. This reflected the seriousness of the issues and the need for high level agreement, because disciplinary action, prosecution and so on could follow from inappropriate use of physical intervention, while lack of an agreed approach could place staff unnecessarily at risk. It was a matter of the utmost importance to secure organisational ownership of the approach to be adopted in both organisations.

2 *Policy on vocational study.* This policy established guidance for managers on deciding whether to release staff for external courses, and was pre-

pared in order to ensure equity across the newly combined service. Consultation was within the service and with personnel. Agreement was with the Joint Service management group who managed all the staff to which the policy applied.

Implementation

The policy will need to be launched and briefed to those who will be affected by it. It should then enter into the day-to-day management of the service. Decide:

1 Do you need a formal launch?
2 Do you need to organise briefing and training for staff and managers? Will different people need different types and levels of training?
3 Does the policy define particular people to take on new responsibilities? If so, they will need to assume these duties.
4 How will you obtain feedback on the effectiveness of the policy?

Now:

1 Define a timetable for implementation, covering the above issues.
2 Agree a frequency for monitoring activities and a review date.

Example from Manchester: establishing a policy and procedures for dealing with allegations of abuse

The preparation of a policy on abuse in Manchester took place under the influence of three incidents:

1 In early 1993 a television documentary addressed the abuse of learning-disabled people in a residential setting. It was discussed by several people in the service.
2 An allegation of abuse required investigation, and this heightened the need for guidance on how to proceed in such cases.
3 The publication of the booklet *It Couldn't Happen Here* (ARC/NAPSAC, 1993) confirmed the need for a framework and focused thinking on the issues.

In 1993 a small working group was established in one area of the city. It consisted of managers and concerned members of staff who recognised the need for policy development. The task seemed huge and the issues difficult. Policies from other areas were obtained and discussed. Links were made, tentatively at first, with other agencies, including the police.

A first draft was produced, and a first consultation took place within the service. It was quite low-key. This led to a second draft and further consultation.

The establishment of the Joint Service in 1994 created a real opportunity for interagency work in policy formulation. It was agreed that the work on abuse was a service priority, which meant that two managers could organise their workload to incorporate the task.

A third draft was produced in April 1994, with a much wider consultation process, which included:

- the Director of Social Services,
- the Trust Chief Executive
- the chair of Social Services Committee
- the chair of the Trust Board
- the Registration and Inspection Unit (Social Services)
- contracts sections
- personnel departments in both organisations
- legal advisers for both organisations

As the document evolved, the need for associated training became apparent. There was a dilemma of whether to wait for a fully ratified policy before starting training, or whether to make a start on training first. The decision was made to begin work on training, as this would help build ownership and understanding of the issues. The social services training section allocated dedicated time to the project.

A three-day course was established by October 1994 and, within 12 months, over 100 staff, including all managers, had attended it.

It was necessary to strike a balance between further redrafting and refinement, and deciding that the policy had reached a point where further rewriting was unnecessary. The final draft document was sent out for its widest consultation in June 1995. The intention was to include as many people and organisations as possible, to ensure that it became a part of everyone's agenda. The circulation of 106 draft copies circulation included:

- social services
- the Mancunian Trust
- all independent providers in the city

- other NHS trusts in the city
- advocacy organisations
- parents' groups
- the police
- colleges and schools
- trade unions
- purchasers of health and social services
- others with a significant stake in the learning disability.

Of these, 45 people or organisations returned their documents with comments so that an extension had to be added to the original consultation period.

Feedback obtained was incorporated into the final document, and the final version was formally tabled and agreed at both the Social Services Committee and the trust board. The policy was launched in May 1996, at an event hosted by Greater Manchester police, with a keynote address from the late Ann Craft, the person in the UK who perhaps did most to raise awareness of the existence of sexual abuse of people with learning disabilities. Over the year April 1996–March 1997 there were four briefing sessions held for statutory and independent sector provider managers attended by over 60 managers from 12 organisations.

The head of service is the lead officer for the policy for all investigations in the city, allowing monitoring of the policy, both in terms of the investigation process and the scale and nature of both alleged and proven abuse.

The actual impact of the policy is less easy to establish, partly because data on allegations and investigations was not separately collected before its advent. However, the clear impression is that there has been an increase in notification of all types of abuse.

Within the Joint Service, there is now a wide consensus that abuse 'can happen here', there is vigilance about it, and clarity about what to do when it is suspected.

Conclusion

Formalising work tasks and procedures ensures bureaucratic control but also provides a developmental function for an organisation. It offers clear roles, expectation and guidance for staff and inculcates, within an organisation, a culture of accountability.

The clarity of purpose and ownership of a policy is critical to ensure its adherence by the target group of staff. Unless briefing or training and later audit of compliance is also undertaken, policies are rarely effective.

This chapter has described good practice in writing policies, consulting on them, their ratification by responsible authorities and the eventual audit of compliance. It uses, as an example, the policy 'Dealing with Allegations of Abuse' – a policy and procedure for health and social care workers – and describes its process from inception to implementation.

Resources

ARC/NAPSAC (1993), *It Could Never Happen Here! The Prevention and Treatment of Sexual Abuse of Adults with Learning Disabilities in Residential Settings*, Chesterfield and Nottingham: Association for Residential Care and National Association for the Protection from Sexual Abuse of Adults and Children with Learning Disabilities.

Brown, H. and Craft, A. (1994), *Thinking the Unthinkable: Papers on Sexual Abuse and People with Learning Difficulties*, London: Family Planning Association.

Learning Disability Services, Manchester (1996), *Policy and Procedures for Health and Social Care Workers Dealing with Allegations of Abuse*, Manchester: Joint Learning Disability Service.

Learning Disability Services, Manchester (1997), *Responding to Violence and Aggression; Including Policy on the Use of Physical Intervention*, Manchester: Joint Learning Disability Service.

North West Training and Development Team (1993), *Abuse, Awareness and Actions: Guidelines for Recognising and Responding to Abuse, Exploitation and Neglect of Adults with Severe Learning Disabilities*, Whalley, Lancashire: North West Training and Development Team.

Part III

Developing the Service

Introduction

The following eight chapters focus on a variety of ways of developing services and their responsiveness. This Part of the book goes beyond the organisational structures and the support of the workforce to consider some of the issues of service content. Drawing, as it does, on our experience in Manchester, this is the most selective part of the book: other aspects could have been chosen. However, the variety in this section again underlines the broad remit of learning disability services, with their responsibility to enhance many aspects of their users' lives.

In Chapter 7, Mike Kellaway and Dave Ruane focus on the radical changes involved in replacing inappropriate services with more and better ones. They draw on their experience of hospital and hostel closure and resettlement, but also draw out more general issues that may help those contemplating other ambitious redevelopments, such as the replacement of day centres.

In Chapter 8 Andrew Pope and his colleagues review issues in facilitating meaningful day care experiences. They present a view that sees no easy answers, but emphasises the importance of moving beyond the day centre model through ensuring clarity about the purpose of daytime activity for each person.

Jane Jolliffe and her colleagues review issues in the development and management of the therapy professions (speech and language therapy, occupational therapy and physiotherapy) in Chapter 9. They also present some of the more innovative work which they have carried out in Manchester and which illustrates the importance of properly integrating their skills and knowledge into services for learning-disabled people.

In recent years there has been a belated recognition of the vulnerability of learning-disabled people to sexual and other abuse, together with a recognition of the scale of the problem. In Chapter 10 Jude Moss and Christine Adcock present a review of these issues and provide a framework for an organisational strategy for effective responses to it, particularly in the continuing support of those who have been victims.

Two chapters follow on behavioural challenges. Chapter 11 by Jean Lally provides a framework for enabling direct care staff to prevent many instances of challenging behaviour by becoming sensitive to distress in service users. In Chapter 12 Mark Burton and Phil Jones address the issue of how to support people who present high levels of challenging behaviour. Their 'clinically managed social care' approach integrates current knowledge about analysis and intervention with behavioural challenges into the day-to-day management of care and support. It is another example of the joint approach that runs throughout this book.

Dave Crier and Mike Petrou have worked to improve the safety of learning-disabled people in the community. Chapter 13, 'Confidence in the Community', describes some of the approaches that they have taken, which are characterised by collaboration with a variety of other organisations.

Finally, Nigel Hoar has pioneered the use of video as a tool in service development. The final chapter in Part III illustrates the promising potential of video at various levels and for a variety of tasks.

7 Redeveloping services
Mike Kellaway and Dave Ruane

Introduction

Much of this book concerns changing the practices within services, or developing new services or extensions to existing services. Sometimes, however, the overall design of a service is so inadequate or inappropriate that it is necessary to completely replace the old service with a new one. This is what is meant by 'redevelopment' here. Examples include:

- the rundown and closure of long-stay hospitals and their replacement with community-based provision
- the closure of hostels and their replacement with supported living in ordinary houses
- the replacement of day centres with a spectrum of alternative provision in the employment, education and recreational, as well as social care, sectors.

This chapter examines the issues that need to be confronted in changing the way in which services are delivered and looks at some of the lessons that can be learnt from Manchester's experience.

Key issues

Towell (1988), in the context of moving from hospital to community provision, identifies three dimensions of a concerted strategy for change:

1 *Establishing the strategic framework*

- policy leadership
- political backing
- principles and vision
- financial policies
- management arrangements
- personnel policies
- staff training and support for innovation

2 *Managing contracting institutions*

- co-ordination arrangements
- staff consultation and participation
- redeployment policies
- individual client relocation
- retrenchment planning
- maintaining quality and morale

3 *Developing local services*

- multi-agency collaboration processes
- establishing shared visions
- participative planning linked to implementation
- individual needs and representation
- locality focus and community involvement
- management and accountability
- staff training and support
- quality safeguards

These all need addressing simultaneously, although there is a sequence of activities, described by Burton (1989) in terms of four overlapping phases:

1 Establishing a vision of what ought to be.
2 Deepening the vision and gaining popular support for it, often through developing 'prefigurative' examples of what might be possible.
3 Developing the capability of the organisation(s) that will have to 'deliver the goods', and
4 Learning both about the means, but also more about the ends, as the vision becomes less of a fantasy and the organisation(s) begin to operate to enable its realisation.

Shared vision and principles: establishing models of service provision

As Towell noted:

> The development of new services should be based on explicit values and a positive vision of the opportunities which should be available to people with learning difficulties. (Towell 1988: 46)

It is crucial to have a sense of what everyone is trying to achieve. Otherwise, the change is likely to bear many of the features of the old model – a process Tyne (1982) described as '"moving away from" rather than "moving toward"', and 'looking over the shoulder'.

A radical, even idealistic, view of an alternative future is helpful, particularly if parts can be validated by already existing 'images of possibility'.

Example

The examples of ENCOR in Nebraska, USA (Thomas, Firth and Kendall, 1978), and early demonstration projects in the UK (for example, Cardiff: Welsh Office, 1978; Bristol: Ward, 1986; and Andover: Felce, 1989) were particularly valuable in making the break with institution-derived models, allowing bold and influential policy documents to be written in the early 1980s (King's Fund, 1980; NWRHA, 1983). This visionary activity was freely drawn upon in many localities.

The first step

One of the hardest things to do for large organisations is to start! The 'big bang' approach to change in social care provision can be effective but will often leave casualties on all sides. The introduction of social services departments in local authorities, after Seebohm in 1970 left many good and talented practitioners rootless and disaffected. Services for some user groups, particularly disabled people, were left to flounder without direction for a number of years. Learning from experience and walking before you can run are useful adages.

Example

Most authorities involved in resettling people from the large institutions have chosen dispersed housing with network teams of support staff. Each network provided a range of housing dependent on the individual needs of service users, and staff were provided throughout 24 hours a day as required.

In some places the massive intellectual, emotional and financial commitment to change that was required of individual families, staff and managers seems to have ground serious redevelopment to a halt – even before it began. Elsewhere, the first resettlement from the large institutions pre-dated, by several years, more comprehensive closure and redevelopment programmes. A number of relatively able men and women were helped to return to ordinary houses with home help, social work and other supports. Mistakes were made, but many lessons were learnt from these early experiences.

The first, more organised, resettlement to staffed houses needed to be successful. Other people living in the institution, and their families and the staff supporting them, needed to see that this vision of community living could work. At each step, the resettlement programme needed to demonstrate clearly the advantages for individuals (and their staff) of returning to their communities. Similarly the resettlement of the first person with multiple disability, the first person with challenging behaviour or mental illness needed to 'succeed' if others were to follow.

The bridging problem

To close and reprovide a service of any size means that, for some time, two services have to be run in parallel. There are therefore dual running costs for the period of redevelopment. For some hospital resettlement schemes (for example, the north-west) this can be for as long as 15 years. A financial framework, including bridging money, is a key requirement. Service users who leave hospitals or hostels inevitably take staff and other resources with them, but in the absence of bridging finance and because of the need to retain some sort of service in the larger establishment, both can often be left underfunded and/or underresourced. With little or no additional funding to redevelop local and comprehensive services, risks were inevitably taken in the hospital and/or hostels.

Involving the affected

Major changes in service delivery require partnership with all the people affected. Ambitious schemes can be derailed in the absence of a consensus alliance among those with an interest in the service (see the postscript to Burton, 1989, for an example). A minimum list of those who need to be involved includes:

1 the people with learning disability and their families
2 the staff and their trade unions
3 the community and its local representatives.

People using services and their families

It is important to recognise the significance of the changes which are being suggested.

For the people who use the service, the change can be considerable.

Example

Some of the people who have resettled from mental handicap hospitals had lived all their life in the large institution. One or two people were actually born there. Some brave and articulate people have described their experience of the institutional life (see, for example, Barron, 1987; Laing, 1992). They describe the waste of their lives in locked and crowded wards and the loss of contact with their extended family and community. There were many caring staff but the institution itself had a brutalising effect on all who lived and worked there. People clearly needed time to adjust to life outside the institution. Sometimes people were expected to make choices about important issues – their future life 'where and who to live with' – when they hadn't had experience of even very basic decision-making.

Other changes might include living in a domestic-scale environment with the different freedoms and pressures that entails or, conversely, being unable to wander freely as they could in the hospital grounds because of danger from traffic.

For families of those using the service, the change can also be a source of uncertainty and threat. Why should they believe the managers and professionals who now say the service which they previously recommended is no longer appropriate, and that life will be better after the redevelopment?

Example

Parents and relatives had been led to believe that the institution was a 'home for life'. Arguments 'that society was unsafe' and that the individual would either be vulnerable to exploitation or a danger to others had been offered by a variety of doctors, nurses and social workers. Families had often struggled to make the difficult decision to let their relative move out of their home to the institution. This trauma and the guilt was resurrected by proposals to close the institution.

Staff and their representatives

Redevelopment can mean a significant change for staff. It can mean completely new working practices, perhaps more isolated, perhaps with more responsibility. It might mean changes of conditions of employment. Even if the particular redevelopment means none of these things, there will be the suspicion that it does.

Example

Many hospital staff had worked in the institution all their careers. It provided their professional development and often a great deal of their social life. Institutions in rural areas provide an employment base for most of the community. The economic implications of the closure of a large hospital on a local village will not be very different from the closure of a coalmine. Many staff who are unqualified and have dependent families cannot afford to travel long distances to work in the new community services.

Staff had been used to working in a supervised setting with line managers on-site. The prospect of working alone in a house on a housing estate in a new neighbourhood, was quite daunting. Night staff had particularly difficult adjustments. Many staff had already adjusted to the challenge of caring for more disabled people with major personal care needs: they now had to deal with the prospect of doing this in ordinary houses with all the constraints of space, stairs, small bathrooms, neighbours, the distance from the bus stop and so on.

Early consultation with staff groups and their trade union representatives is essential. There may be few options available. Clear and prompt communication is critical if the cooperation and goodwill of staff is to be maintained.

Communities and their representatives

Much of the social revolution in the care of disabled people has been achieved under the banner of 'care in the community'. Many critics have decried this, questioning 'What care?', 'What community?'. What has not been realised generally is the depth of the implications of inclusive living in the community for ordinary citizens as well as for service users and providers.

Communities near an existing service can lose:

- **A source of employment.** Hospitals were often located in rural areas where other employment prospects are poor. In Victoria, Australia, the state government actually carried out social impact studies (cf. Finterbusch *et al.*, 1983) to establish the consequences for the local economy of closure of large isolated institutions and to plan for alternative sources of work.
- **A social focus.** A service that groups people together is visible and can act as a focus for caring actions. While these may be patronising, it would be a shame to lose the possibility of maintaining this impulse and working to transform it into a more inclusive form of social solidarity.

Communities with little prior experience of people with significant disability can feel threatened. It is incumbent on everyone working in learning disability services to advocate for community inclusion (unlike the senior

---

Example

Most resettlement from hospitals and hostels has been achieved with no opposition from tenants or neighbourhood groups. The model of most resettlement, into ordinary sized housing with staff support, has made it difficult for neighbours to rally opposition. Planning permission has not been necessary, so notice has not been given to neighbours. It is clearly important that local councillors, who are involved, understand and are committed to the process.

It does not seem helpful to ask neighbours 'permission' to move people into a house. The rights of disabled people to take and use all parts of the community cannot be compromised before they have even moved in! It is important that staff help individuals to be 'good neighbours' and that this begins as the delivery van arrives. Complaints and concerns expressed by neighbours about noise or unusual behaviour need to be addressed promptly and with sensitivity.

professional who actively opposed a staffed house next door!), and to use every opportunity to inform, explain and debunk the myths that can evolve. The principled leadership of elected representatives and other prominent people in the community is to be sought and cultivated.

Building a coalition for change

It is helpful to understand organisational and social change in terms of a political metaphor.

For social change to take place and for its gains to be maintained, requires the mobilisation of a social movement. Positive change in the learning disability arena can be understood in relation to the emergence of alliances that cohere around key ideological positions (Lewis, Kagan and Burton, 1995). Recent changes in the life experiences of learning-disabled people in Western countries have involved diverse elements in coalitions for change. For example, the establishment of early intervention programmes, in the 1960s and 1970s came about through a broad alliance that subsequently shaped much of the agenda of the system through the 1970s and 1980s. This alliance is best regarded as a fairly loose coalition between parents, professionals, managers, academics, legislators and advocates which had a general consensus about the desirability of development, opportunity and community living. Such ideologies, when consistently promoted, take on concrete forms in the shape of practices, policies and services. The resulting service models provide images of possibility, but also constrain the imagination of how to implement the rather abstract philosophy. There are, of course, tensions in such alliances. The constituent parties have different interests and, moreover, the achievements of the movement (as services) engender particular identities and commitments. Over time, however, the philosophy has evolved to encompass increasingly sophisticated and theorised notions of living in the community with provision of service and non-service supports to do so. However, such coalitions for progressive and principled change have their strongest bases in the service system itself and are therefore vulnerable to destabilisation from forces transmitted through the power structures.

In promoting redevelopment there is a need to build such alliances, and to maintain and renew them. However, as indicated above, this is not to impose a 'one true way' on the various stakeholder groups, but to learn together, continuously adjusting assumptions, theories and models, and improving services.

Contraction/closure of services

The process of closing down existing provision needs care. Consider, for a moment, the implicit messages of a redevelopment scheme to both the staff and service users who still remain with the service that is being run down. On the one hand, they are being asked to remain, to continue as before, and to maintain standards, but at the same time the clear message is that this service is no longer wanted. Maintaining morale is critical here, and this is perhaps best done in a culture of openness and honesty, where staff can be involved in decision-making, can confront some of the dilemmas facing the service, and can provide the benefit of their experience to the change process.

Example: hospital closure

Brockhall Hospital in Lancashire closed ward by ward, unit by unit. To some extent, the order of closure was determined by the layout of the heating and other utility systems. Where possible, the people living in each ward were resettled as it closed but, because people were returning to a variety of localities and in small groups, some people had to move within the hospital, or even to a nearby hospital, before they could return home. While nobody was happy about these 'chequerboard moves' there was a general commitment (within the hospital and in the receiving districts) to minimising them, and the hospital closed according to schedule, releasing funds for the support of people in their new communities.

Example: hostel closure

A hostel where 24 young people lived was due to close. It had been built in the form of four self-contained 'houses' with their own facilities but, in true institutional style, there was a central kitchen that provided meals. The respite care service, based on one of the 'houses', first changed its base to a community house, under the management of the small housing network that already existed. Then the kitchen closed; the cooks were regraded as support staff, and each house became 'self catering'. The first group of three people moved out to their new home, and the remaining people in their house moved into a staff flat, sharing staff with one of the remaining 'houses'. This meant that half the original accommodation was now empty, and this was taken over by the new tenants who took responsibility for half of the building running costs. The rest of the closure followed.

At the same time, a decisive approach should be maintained towards the closure of parts of the service. The key here is to ensure that resources are released promptly, but without compromising the support of those who remain. This means having a coherent plan for the closure of elements of the service and the release of funds.

Closure and redevelopment are not easy. As the examples above show, some people suffer temporary disruption. This is why the management of the process must combine both clarity about values and goals, *and* efficiency and determination to ensure that change happens in as smooth and dignified manner as possible.

Don't put up what you cannot take down

That which replaces the old might itself show inadequacies in the future: managers are not clairvoyant and, while they can act in good faith, they cannot anticipate every possible problem. One manager used to show slides of the demolition of Manchester's high-rise deck access housing disasters of the 1960s to make this point. The message is: try to create new provision that lends itself to alteration.

Example: compatibility – Naomi's experience

Naomi moved out of a hostel into a house with two other people. At the time, it was recognised that the grouping was not ideal and, over the next few months, she became more and more withdrawn, preferring to sit on the landing rather than in the lounge with the others. Staff tried a variety of strategies to help her feel more at ease in the house, but had little success. A visiting support worker did some useful focused work to help her engage in purposeful activities which she enjoyed, but it proved difficult to maintain this impetus between visits. Problems also became apparent with the house which was shoddily built and noisy.

Eventually it was decided that the three people should move. A vacancy became available in another house and Naomi moved there. Her co-tenants moved together to a new home. From the start Naomi settled well, and the work by the visiting worker took off, leading to a reduction of withdrawal and thereby transforming Naomi's day-to-day experience.

In the above example it was relatively easy to move to a different house: it makes sense to leave housing purchase and management to housing departments and housing associations. Care providers do not have a good record as landlords. Service users can have greater flexibility to move on or reconfigure if they rent their own property.

Manchester's experience of redeveloping residential services

Over the last 30 years the pattern of care for learning-disabled people has changed dramatically. In 1970 there were over 400 admissions, both long-term and short-term, from Manchester to the large mental handicap hospitals. Today Cranage, Mary Dendy, Brockhall and Royal Albert are already closed and Calderstones, which in its heyday had a patient population of 2000, is set to close by 1998.

From the mid-1960s Manchester had developed a capacity within the city to accommodate people with a learning disability. There were seven hostels for adults and three for children. The adult hostels did not care for people with profound or multiple disability. The children's homes, on the other hand, provided for a much greater range of people. There are, today, no hostels for learning-disabled people in the city. This pattern of change from an institutional model of care to an individual model of care has been, or is being, replicated throughout the country.

This period of change and upheaval, of resistance and triumph, success and failure was crammed into a very short period. Many service users and a number of staff have experienced this revolution in social care. The test for its success will be if the real experience of quality of life has changed for service users and families and whether managers and staff can sustain and protect services into the future.

Resettlement from the hospitals

In 1980 many learning-disabled people lived in large institutions, usually built by the Victorians and often a long way from their town of origin. Most institutions had been developed either by philanthropists, by the old Poor Law boards or by followers of the eugenic movement. Over the years, they had been managed both inside and outside of the National Health Service. All were segregated from the rest of society. Inmates were grouped together in large numbers and had all their needs met on-site. Those services which were provided more locally were developed in the 1950s and 1960s and took the form of hostels or day centres. The model was to congregate people with 'similar' disabilities in large groups within, but isolated from, the rest of the community.

Manchester used several large institutions to place people with a learning disability prior to 1985. There were 483 Mancunians identified in the hospitals in Table 7.1.

In the early 1980s it had been established that Calderstones Hospital would be the catchment hospital for Manchester.

Table 7.1   Manchester's resettlement task, by hospital

Hospital	Number of Mancunians
Green Lane Children's Home, Ormskirk	1
Swinton House, Salford	12
Offerton House, Stockport	18
Royal Albert, Lancaster	22
Brockhall, Blackburn	150
Calderstones, Whalley	280
Total	483

Example: Calderstones

Calderstones was a large institution built in rural Lancashire during the First World War. It was originally commissioned to care for wounded soldiers but subsequently became a county learning disability hospital. Because it was a self-contained community, people rarely left the hospital to access local resources. The hospital site had its own church where religious services were held for all denominations. In addition, the hospital had its own fire station with members of staff creating a part-time fire service, its own farm, which produced a whole range of home-grown produce and a range of livestock, and its own school. Workshops and daytime occupation centres were developed. If people became ill and required an operation, they went to a general hospital but, as soon as appropriate, they were discharged back to Calderstones for convalescence. Within the grounds, shops were developed, often with stock from within the hospital; there were also a tailor's shop, a cobbler and dressmakers. The hospital dentist held dental surgeries in which patients often had total extractions after biting themselves, other patients or staff. The total needs of the patient population was provided on-site, and people often spent their whole lives within the confines of the institution. As the hospital also had its own mortuary and graveyard, some people grew up and died within the confines of the hospital and never ventured out of its grounds

Community Care legislation and strategy for hospital closure

The early acceptance of the shared vision of the Model District Services ordinary life principles forced authorities to shift their thinking away from institutional and towards community-based services. This meant a radical change in how learning-disabled people were supported. To take the city of Manchester as an example, service users had either lived with their family, lived in one of seven 24-place hostels spread throughout the city, or were transported 30 miles or more to the large institutions throughout the region.

From the early 1980s new community-based multidisciplinary teams began to support learning-disabled people, locally, either living at home with parents or in one of the local hostels. The main aim was to be proactive, offer the support required locally and thereby reduce or eliminate the need for admission to Calderstones.

In 1984 representatives of health and local authority services in Manchester planned with hospital and regional officers to develop a ten-year strategy for the rundown and closure of the large hospitals in the North Western Regional Health Authority and, later, the Mersey Regional Health Authority. Manchester agreed that the strategy needed to be a city-wide venture. Although each district health authority would take responsibility for resettling their own named individuals, the programme would continue to be coordinated on a city-wide basis and led by social services in a programme lasting ten years outlined below in Table 7.2. The process was prolonged and drawn out due to Manchester City Council's and the three district health authorities' determination that the scheme should incur no extra cost to local services.

Table 7.2 Manchester's resettlement task, by year

Year ending	Estimated number of Mancunians remaining in hospital	Mancunian hospital population (%)
31.3.88	381	78.9
31.3.89	330	68.3
31.3.90	280	58.0
31.3.91	232	48.0
31.3.92	185	38.3
31.3.93	139	28.8
31.3.94	95	29.7
31.3.95	52	10.8

A Model District Service

The North Western Regional Health Authority set out criteria for interagency planning on the basis of individual need in its policy paper *A Model District Service* (NWRHA, 1982). Manchester was fortunate in having this document – which was the envy of many local and health authorities throughout the UK – to shape the future provision of care for learning-disabled people. The document laid down a philosophy of care that should be local, comprehensive and integrated. Care should be provided in small homes, which should accommodate no more than six people.

Infrastructure

Manchester had already resettled 26 people prior to the ten-year programme commencing in 1987. The funding for this group provided the opportunity for the local authority and three district health authorities to 'front-load' the cost of the new services, including some of the early infrastructure and professional costs.

The resettlement process

Community learning disability nurses and social workers were employed as resettlement officers in North, Central and South Manchester. Each district had a list of names of residents, and these resettlement officers were directed to carry out joint assessments of the individuals concerned and attend individual planning meetings held at the hospitals. Finding people with established relationships or establishing other means of testing compatibility was a very difficult process. Calderstones converted several staff houses on the hospital perimeter and some staff flats to patient accommodation to provide experience of domestic-type housing and to test for group compatibility. There were many obstacles to this process – clarity about individuals' capability, compatibility, medical history and current medical information was patchy.

The hospital and hospital staff put much effort into preparing people for resettlement. Resettlement teams of social workers and nurses took people to meet others who had already moved out, to see their new neighbourhood and to be involved in the choice of house and furnishings. Hospital staff often accompanied people resettling throughout the transitional period: some were seconded to Manchester for several months, and some transferred to local jobs in the city. This strategy was encouraged in the RHA document, *Positive Futures for Staff*, which demonstrated the need for staff to move out of the hospital with patients to avoid creating an enormous redundancy problem on hospital closure. It was also important that skilled staff were not lost to the service.

During the financial year 1990–91 escalating costs and national pay agreements for local authority staff led to a shift in direction. The social services department began to negotiate placements with the independent sector and non-profit-making agencies, rather than resettle to directly provided services.

To date, over 200 Mancunians have returned from the long-stay hospitals to lead more valued lifestyles in their local communities. The majority live in a variety of houses, flats and bungalows, comprising local authority housing stock and housing association properties. Twelve people have died now – a much lower death rate than anticipated from hospital rates. The financial resources attached to the support for those people has been reinvested to provide community-based services for other people who would have previously been placed in long-stay hospitals.

Over the years of the resettlement programme it became increasingly obvious that additional skills were required to support certain individuals whose behaviour was difficult to manage. This led to the development of clinically managed sites in North and Central Manchester (see further Chapter 11).

At a very early stage, every organisation concerned with the redevelopment of services had agreed that any money provided must ultimately go into developing services for all service users, irrespective of whether they come from the region's hospitals, hostels or family homes from within the city. In 1990 the resettlement networks were combined with the mainstream networks established to support people from the hostels and who had moved on from their families. This avoided a 'two-tier' service, for those with a resettlement 'dowry' and those without.

Adult placement

A significant number of people have been resettled into adult placements from the large institutions. This scheme recruits individuals and families to take a learning-disabled person into their homes and provide for their ongoing needs. The adult placement carer receives financial recompense, support and training from the social services department.

Hostel replacement

Manchester social services department established hostels for learning-disabled people in the 1960s. By 1980 there were four adult hostels – three purpose-built to accommodate 25 people each and one a converted old house also accommodating 24 people. There were also three children's homes. The hostels have been described as 'wards at the end of streets'. The model of care was necessarily institutional, with set meal-times, bath nights, TV lounges and group outings, but staff worked hard to individualise care within the environment. It was easier for family and friends to keep in touch with their relatives in the hostel than if they were placed in one of the hospitals out of town. Although each had developed differently, the adult hostels were mostly staffed by local people, female staff outnumbered male and staff were employed on manual grades. The children's homes cared for more physically disabled and profoundly learning-disabled young people. They were more likely to have qualified managers and staff were often younger and male. By 1980 staff had been recruited on professional grades. All hostels had cooks, cleaners and driver-handymen. Residents and their families tended to view the hostels as 'homes for life'.

Because the demand for respite care had increased as the department sought to shift provision away from the large hospital, each hostel provided a number of short-term care beds. By 1985 there were 20 such beds, used by over 100 families. However, it became increasingly evident that providing short-term care in the hostel was disruptive to the long-term residents. Furthermore, the population of the children's homes was rapidly growing up and it began to prove very difficult to move them on to the adult hostels which were mostly full and which, in any case, had great difficulty in caring for multiply disabled people.

The pressure to change the model of care from hostels was due to a variety of factors:

1 *A Model District Service* was published in 1982.
2 The dissemination of clearly articulated philosophies (normalisation/ social role valorisation/the 'ordinary life' model) through the value-based training which had originated in Scandinavia and North America, was taking hold in the UK, particularly in the north-west, by the mid-1980s.
3 The resettlement programme agreed between Manchester City Council, the three district health authorities and the regional health authority began in 1984, and care was being provided in ordinary housing. The Social Services Committee was determined that there should not be a two-tier service – one for local people and one for resettled people.
4 The physical condition of a number of the hostels, which had suffered years of cutbacks on maintenance, now required urgent action.
5 The vision of individual officers and members of the Social Services Committee and a local housing association led to the development of the Lapwing Lane Scheme. A very sheltered housing unit and a number

of flats and houses were built in a corner of one of the smarter suburbs of South Manchester. Accommodation was made available to older people who needed warden support, young families and individuals with learning disabilities who, for the first time, had staff support in their own home according to need, often through 24 hours.

6   The specialist social workers within the department had already returned 26 people from the long-stay hospital before the resettlement programme began. These people were supported in ordinary houses, mostly living in groups of three or four, with home help and social work support. In 1982 special domiciliary carer teams were established to provide this support. The department was developing its expertise in managing care in dispersed housing.

The first hostel to close was a converted doctor's residence. It needed major work and was unlikely to meet the minimum standards being established by the Registered Homes Act 1988. The decision to close the building and relocate the residents to ordinary housing was pre-empted by problems with the drains and the boiler! At the same time, the social services department was closing its 59 family group homes, which accommodated four or six children each. The officer leading the closure of Summerhill accessed some of these and also negotiated tenancies with the housing department.

A report, *Redevelopment of Residential Services for Mentally Handicapped People* went to the Social Services Committee in January 1991. It outlined the task of closing six hostels and relocating residents into ordinary housing. Some hostel residents would move into adult placement – a new scheme which recruited host families to provide long-term care. The majority, however, would be supported by networks of staff working flexibly through 24 hours.

North, South and Central Manchester established joint planning groups between the health authorities and social services. Families and individuals were consulted, and individual planning processes took place. At the beginning of the hostel closure programme the housing department provided tenancies. There were also some ex-family group homes available, which were reopened. Some properties were commissioned from housing associations; this was particularly necessary to accommodate physically disabled people. Staff from the adult hostels were transferred from manual grade to a professional grade before they moved into the community. Consultation, training and counselling was necessary to reassure staff that they would be able to manage care in dispersed sites. Because the first group to move out was often critical to the programme, staff, at that early stage, would continue to receive management from the hostel managers. The improved quality of the environment in which they worked, the immediate progress of service users in their new homes, the improved staffing levels and greater opportunity to use the community all helped staff to overcome their concerns about working away from direct management support.

The changes in working practice that the department required of staff were considerable. Most were managing finances and the administration of medication for the first time. In the hostels, they had not generally been required to 'sleep in'. Waking-night staff – available to provide care through the night – were working alone for the first time. Issues about travelling to and from houses in different parts of the city, security and personal safety were high on the agenda.

Partway through the redevelopment programme, the management of the process was centralised in order to ensure that deadlines were met. It had become increasingly difficult to locate accessible properties of sufficient size to accommodate three or four service users. The pressure to close particular hostels, often due to failing fire safety standards or minimum standards of repair and decoration led to the decision to combine the residents of two hostels in the last hotel to close – a situation mirrored in the closure of the large north-west hospitals.

The final hostel with 11 residents, all of whom were multiply disabled, closed in 1994. The department had negotiated an arrangement with a housing association to demolish the hostel and build very sheltered housing in the form of five bungalows. Care was to be provided by a voluntary organisation. The redevelopment of the hostels programme had to be done within the hostel budget and was always going to be a difficult task. At the end of the programme compromises had to be made involving residents moving several times in three years and living in adjacent built bungalows.

As a result of the hostel redevelopment programme and resettlement from hospitals, a variety of provision has been developed:

- *Houses with 24-hour waking support.* At least one of these was required in each of the neighbourhood networks. These support individuals in the greatest need, often with profound multiple disability or challenging behaviour. Staff are on duty through 24 hours a day, including waking night duty. Many houses have double cover all or most of the time.
- *Houses with 24-hour support with sleep-in.* These properties have staff available until service users wish to retire at 11 pm or midnight. The staff on late duty then sleep in, on-site, in case service users require support during the night. If disturbed for more than a reasonable amount of time, arrangements are made for a disturbed sleep-in allowance and/or time taken back in lieu.

- *Houses with waking hours support.* These sites house service users who have developed skills, through training and risk-taking packages, that permit support to be withdrawn when they retire. As part of the risk-taking packages, telephones are either linked to staffed houses or community alarm systems have been installed.
- *Minimum support houses.* These offer support at key times in people's lives to assist with budgeting, medication and development or maintenance of independent living skills.

  One hostel had placed six people, needing very limited support, in separate flats within a low-level block. Initial efforts to have support provided by a tenant living rent-free did not work out but, even with one staff member on-site, throughout 24 hours, it has been an economic option that, as a formal evaluation study has shown, gives a good balance of support with independence.
- *Adult placement.* This is a scheme, now managed outside the Joint Service, in which people live with host families.

Review of models

Due to rising costs in service delivery, the way in which the service is provided had to be reviewed. This meant that every property and every single service user's needs had to be examined carefully to make more effective use of staff. This has resulted in a dramatic reduction in the amount of staff time used across the service. Particular attention was made to targeting staff support to the times when it was really required by service users. An outcome of this has been a reduction in the number of double-cover sites, as well as an increased clarity about what staff are actually expected to do when on duty.

The development of a more flexible workforce has also led to the service becoming more effective and efficient in its delivery. The move has been from a workforce which was predominantly working full-time to one which comprises a mix of full-time staff and part-timers, the latter working flexible shifts. Peripatetic staff teams, covering more than one network, have also been developed to stand in for staff unavailable for work.

Recouping resources?

A major problem in the hospital closure programme has been the disposal of the site. The institutions were as big as small villages; Calderstones had its own railway line, mortuary, fire station and church. Little of this real estate could be disposed of before the completion of resettlement. Currently, under 300 people live at Calderstones but 1500 staff remain and over 500 of these are not providing a direct care service. The cost of upkeep and of staff involved has constrained what is available to resettle individuals. The freeing of capital at closure never seemed to realise the expected amounts.

This situation was worse in the city. The hostels had been poorly maintained for many years and could not even be sold to the new legion of independent providers. Those that were sold did not realise a large amount of money. Regulations about capital receipts and the local authorities' own organisational rules meant that none of this money found its way back to services for disabled people.

Staffing

In the late 1980s recruitment in Manchester was principally directed towards people who could demonstrate a clear understanding of positive social values at interview. We ended up with articulate, young, educated people, many of whom were incomers to Manchester. Afterwards we realised that we needed more variety of skills, ages and interests. The people to be supported were often middle-aged or elderly. A major task was clearly homemaking. For service users the staff are their main link with the community and it helps if they are part of, and know, that community. The interests of service users are wide and varied. Staff with an interest in ballroom dancing, gardening, organ music and so on will promote that variety and individuality.

Everyone who lived in the hospital and hostels had waking-night support, whether they needed it or not. Withdrawal of night staff could be very difficult. We all knew people who stayed awake to keep the night staff company!

Institutions had their working days and nights divided into shifts which were easily covered by full-time staff. The new model of care, on dispersed sites, had key times which are more easily covered by part-time staff who also provide managers with much greater flexibility.

Managers will take time to settle into their new role. Managing support in a number of houses, at a distance, is all about managing risk and having systems. Looking back, how did we manage without them? Each network house has the following:

- *A personal record system*: 19 sheets for each individual, comprising a personal profile, appointments with doctor, dentist, chiropodist, timetable of regular activity each week, inventory of personal possessions, family contact number and so on.

- *A list of standards*: For example, 'All tenants will have the opportunity to go out twice each week without other disabled people' and their method of audit.
- *A number of policies/procedures*: These cover risk management, missing person procedure, administering medication and so on.
- *A recording system*:
  - handover books
  - financial accounting
  - medication charts

Conclusion

Service redevelopment can be worth the effort, although such upheavals are likely to have costs (both human and financial) as well as benefits. In Manchester, the hospital and hostel redevelopments have led to:

- a development of local resources once concentrated in a few sites
- the more efficient use of resources previously tied up in institutional buildings and their maintenance
- access to more generic sources of finance, such as housing benefit
- the development of more individualised and responsive models of care and support.

Getting this far has taken considerable commitment and vision, as well as effective management of resources, staff and processes over many years. A great deal has been learned on the way, but there is much more to learn as we continue trying to create services that authentically support people in 'real community living'.

References and resources

Barron, D. (1987), 'Locked away', *Community Living* 1 (2), 8–9.

Burton, M. (1989), *Australian Intellectual Disability Services: Experiments in Social Change*, Working Paper in Building Community Strategies 1, London: King's Fund College.

Carpenter, M. (1994), *Normality is Hard Work: Trade Unions and the Politics of Community Care*, London: Lawrence and Wishart.

Cocks, E. (1994), *Encouraging a Paradigm Shift in Services for People with Disabilities*, Social Research and Development Monograph No 9, Joondalup, Western Australia: Edith Cowan University; Centre for the Development of Human Resources.

DHSS (1983), *Care in the Community*, HC(83)6 and LAC(83)5, London: DHSS.

Dluhy, M.L. (1990), *Building Coalitions in the Human Services*, Newbury Park and London: Sage.

Felce, D. (1989), *Staffed Housing for Adults with Severe or Profound Mental Handicaps: The Andover Project*, Kidderminster, BIMH Publications.

Finterbusch, K., Llewellyn, L. and Wolf, C. (1983), *Social Impact Assessment Methods*, Beverley Hills, California: Sage.

Goffman, E. (1968), *Asylums: Essays on the Social Situation of Mental Patients and Other Inmates*, Harmondsworth: Penguin.

Kanter, R.M., Stein, B.A. and Jick, T.D. (1992), *The Challenge of Organizational Change: How Companies Experience it and Leaders Guide it*. New York: Free Press.

King's Fund Centre (1980), *An Ordinary Life: Comprehensive Locally-based Residential Services for Mentally Handicapped People*, London: King's Fund Centre.

Korman, N. and Glennerster, H. (1990), *Hospital Closure: A Political and Economic Study*, Milton Keynes: Open University Press.

Laing, J. (1992), *Fifty Years in the System*, London: Corgi.

Lewis, S., Kagan, C. and Burton, M. (1995), *Families, Work and Empowerment: Coalitions for Social Change*, IOD Occasional Papers, 5/95, Manchester: IOD Research Group.

North Western Regional Health Authority (1982), *Services for People Who are Mentally Handicapped: A Model District Service*, Manchester: NWRHA.

North Western Regional Health Authority (1983), *Mental Handicap Funding Policy*, Manchester: NWRHA.

NWDT (1989), *Evaluation of the Regional Resettlement Benefits Group*, Whalley: NWDT.

Parston, G. (ed.) (1986), *Managers as Strategists*, London: King Edward's Hospital Fund.

Pettigrew, A., Ferlie, E. and McKie, L. (1992), *Shaping Strategic Change: Making Change in Large Organisations – The Case of the National Health Service*, London: Sage.

Thomas, D., Firth, H. and Kendall, A. (1978), *ENCOR – A Way Ahead*, CMH Enquiry Paper 6, London: Campaign for Mentally Handicapped People.

Towell, D. (1988), 'Managing strategic change in services for people with learning disabilities', in D. Towell (ed.), *An Ordinary Life in Practice*, London: King's Fund.

Tyne, A. (1982), 'Community care and mentally handicapped people', in A. Walker (ed.), *Community Care: The Family, the State and Social Policy*, Oxford: Blackwell.

Ward, L. (1986), 'From hospital to ordinary houses, ordinary streets', *The Health Service Journal*, 1 May, 601.

Weisbord, M.R. and Janoff, S. (1995), *Future Search: An Action Guide to Finding Common Ground in Organizations and Communities*, San Francisco, California: Berrett Koehler.

Welsh Office (1978), *NIMROD: Report of a Joint Working Party on the Provision of a Community Based Mental Handicap Service in South Glamorgan*, Cardiff: Welsh Office.

8 Developing days

Andrew Pope
with contributions by Ian Crabtree, Iain Larkin and
Debbie Windley

Introduction

For the past 20 or more years, day service provision for learning-disabled people has been dominated by two ideas, both of which were central to the influential report of the National Development Group *Day Services for Mentally Handicapped Adults* (NDG, 1977).

On the one hand there has been a shift away from 'work training' to a broader-based social education model (which has been seen as encompassing work skills and necessary work-related social skills). At the same time there has been an increasing impetus towards the use of 'ordinary community facilities'.

The National Development Group's report also made reference to 'special care' facilities within the day service setting. Indeed, much local authority day service provision currently has a 'special care' component, providing services for those people with multiple physical disabilities and/ or sensory deficits, and for people whose behaviour is judged to be particularly challenging.

In many areas, health service involvement in day services has been solely on the basis of individual practitioners having input on a case-work basis, devising and supporting programmes with individual service users, often those placed in special care sections and, personal experience suggests, often in conditions of 'crisis'.

The escalation in both the total volume and individual severity of need which has accompanied the hospital closure programme has put considerable pressure on services. As early as 1971, the White Paper, *Better Services for the Mentally Handicapped*, recognised that a move from institutional to community-based care involved, as its necessary corollary, a considerable increase in day service provision. At that stage, the target set for the early 1990s was for 75 000 day service places. Although provision climbed steadily until the mid-1980s, that process has now slowed, leaving targets still unmet.

In addition to supporting those returning to local communities as a part of the hospital closure programme, day services have been an important factor in preventing admission to long-term care. This is particularly true for those people who challenge services and those with multiple disabilities. As a result, further pressure is put on provision. At the same time, in many areas, there was considerable financial pressure on the 'ordinary community facilities' which people were to make use of. For example, over the last ten years, Manchester has suffered financial pressures on everything from leisure services to adult education places as a result of reductions in central government funding of local authorities and the capping of local taxation.

Even if targets were to be met, there remains the problem of what day services are supposed to do. The goal of supported living in ordinary housing is a reasonably clear and consensual goal for residential/home-making services. It is less obvious either what a culturally equivalent model of day services might be for our most disabled citizens, or what supports would have to be put in place to realise such a goal.

Key issues and practical guidance

Clarifying purposes

It is difficult to provide a good service without being clear about what it is trying to achieve. First we must determine what day services mean to the key groups of people concerned – to service users, their families, to staff within the service, and to people in any outside agencies involved. Services tend to have both explicit and (to borrow Emerson's term) 'latent' functions and missions. Both need to be addressed if there is to be consensus on purposes.

Do we mean to offer work, education, respite, a social gathering or leisure activities? Can these functions be reconciled, and how are priorities to be balanced when different functions appear to be in conflict? Would a negative, isolated experience of low-paid employment be preferable to a familiar social situation in a day centre? How would that preference be modified were the former to be available five days a week and the latter for only two?

If a statement of purpose enables us to balance different needs, it must also be achievable. This is an era of sustained mass unemployment coupled with an expansion of casual, low-paid employment. These changes bring into question whether full employment for people with severe learning disabilities is either achievable or desirable (Richards, 1983).

Towards a possible model

To have reservations about the possibility of full supported employment for all learning-disabled people is not to deny that real work should be a central plank in the mission of daytime supports. There is an urgent need for a greater commitment of resources, planning and innovation in this area in order to expand all types of opportunity from supported employment to social businesses and entrepreneurial ventures in the form of workshops and retail outlets.

Taking our cue from critiques of lifelong paid employment, it seems possible to begin piecing together an integrationist model in which work is seen as one important aspect of a lifetime's activity with fluid movement between employment, community organisation, education and active self-defining leisure and recreation.

Such a model might offer an analogue to the model of supported living in ordinary houses by offering access to a normatively valued activity, and seems to offer a potential *rapprochement* between the needs of service users and their families.

Support versus readiness

People with severe learning disabilities do not need to be 'ready' to live in ordinary houses, but rather require the appropriate supports to do so. The same argument can be applied to daytime opportunities. Unfortunately, day service provision of all sorts is still generally dominated by a philosophy of 'readiness' rather than 'support' – although some progress has been made in the implementation of 'support' models in the field of supported employment. Perhaps its persistence is connected to the difficulty in identifying plausible models for ordinary daytime living that do not depend on a utopian image of full employment. At the same time, the traditional day centre, with its multiple functions, serving the needs of multiple stakeholders (including families and staff), still exerts an influence on service design comparable to that exerted by the institution before the decisive break with tradition was made through the introduction of the staffed housing model.

Thinking 'outside day services'

Perhaps the most important key to developing a more inclusive and user-responsive model is to abandon the image of the day service, and instead work back from the normative and valued analogues. Applying the support philosophy to them allows the development of alternative models of daytime support. Only once this has been done is it necessary to consider whether the logistics of providing support means compromise on issues of integration and individualisation (see Examples 1 and 2 opposite).

Both examples demonstrate the need for detailed and specific planning – for instance, the identification of an appropriate college course, liaison with potential tutors regarding student needs, initiating and coordinating a 'buddy' scheme with fellow students. Establishing and supporting a cooperatively run cafe is a much bigger undertaking, but it can be approached through detailed planning about appropriate premises, relationships between the individual and other cooperative members, task analysis, skill training and support.

Community resources

If the service is to be based on, or make use of, ordinary community resources, these must be identified properly. Some areas are relatively rich in diverse resources, while others have little to draw upon. Just what resources do you intend to use? How many people will use them? For how long? What will they do there? Unless you address these issues in some detail, planning will be vague and services will fail to produce any real integration.

Staff identity

Likewise, thought needs to be paid to the identity of staff. What skills, knowledge and experience will be important for these people, carrying out these tasks, in these places? What other identities might staff need, for example what age, gender and ethnic mix would best help pave the way for acceptance and involvement? If we are helping older men to take part in an a bowls club, then perhaps older men and women would be the best choice for staffing. If the needs are complex, then the mix of professional knowledge and skill within the staff group will need to be considered.

Example 1
A person who has autism attends a further education college for a part-day.

Pattern of day	Resources needed
Travel from home by public transport	Escort with detailed knowledge of person and appropriate skills
Shopping and coffee	
College class	Courses available at appropriate level – tutors briefed on person's needs and prepared to be flexible. Additional support in class, at least for the first few sessions
Lunch	Possibility of developing a 'buddy' system for lunchtime
College class	As for morning class
Swimming	Escort to baths and accompaniment in changing rooms and pool
Travel home	As with the morning

Example 2
The same person supported in working in a cooperatively run cafe

Pattern of day	Resources needed
Travel from home by public transport	Escort with detailed knowledge of person and with appropriate skills
Arrival at workplace	Premises, support staff and start-up
Preparation and cleaning	monies, a planned work routine with a distribution of varied tasks between co-op members
Visit to wholesalers	
Serving	
Washing up	
Doing the books/cashing up	
Visiting bank	
Coffee	
Travel home	As with the morning

Degree of specialisation

Some services try to 'be all things to all people', while others limit their remit. It is important to be clear about the degree of specialisation for each service. Specialisation can refer to service user characteristics and needs (for example, a service for resettled older women or a service for people with additional sensory impairments), and to the content of the day (for example, a work orientation, a developmental orientation or a social and leisure orientation). Some advantages and disadvantages of specialisation according to service user need include:

Pros	Cons
• Commonality of need allows aspects of service design to be consistent – for example, recruitment and training of staff.	• Potentially isolating and inward-looking.
• May allow better matching of staffing level to need.	• Danger of overly uniform approach and narrowness of focus.
• Enables clarity of mission.	• If a high-need service, stress may be a problem.
• Tend to be on a small scale which facilitates community usage and innovation.	• Danger of deskilling the wider service.
• May allow people with highest level of need to receive most focused supports.	• May be stigmatising.
	• Can become a way of not addressing problems within the wider service. Vulnerable to staff changes, changes in funding.

Location and localisation

- Where are services to be based?
- What is the proposed catchment area of the service?
- What is the scale of the proposed service?
- Should the service be in a residential area or among workplaces?

Even if services are not building-based, the catchment area and scale of any proposed service clearly needs consideration, as does some facility for staff coordination, meetings, and so on: what will happen when staff are sick, or outside activities or events are cancelled?

Anticipate pressures

Not all problems can be anticipated, but by identifying the likely pressures on a service, problems can be avoided that might otherwise emerge later. Pressures can arise both from within the service and from outside.

Internal pressures

Small services in particular are likely to be vulnerable to internal pressures – for example:

- Staff sickness can present problems, particularly if several staff are ill at the same time: arrangements for obtaining cover should be made.
- Staff leave needs a degree of management to avoid clashes and also to ensure staff actually take their allowance.
- Arranging service coordination and training can be difficult in a service with limited resources, most of which are tied up in supporting service users: the service must be resourced to allow these tasks to be carried out and organised so that they do happen, rather than allowing things to drift along so that pressures accumulate.
- Stress can be an issue, particularly where staff constantly work with high levels of need: it makes sense to build in ways of preventing stress.

External pressures

External pressures can arise from various sources, for example:

- Pressure to accept more referrals to the service can build up, particularly if there are shortfalls elsewhere in the system. It is worth defining clearly the capacity of the service and the criteria for entry.
- All services, and particularly pilot projects, are potentially vulnerable to funding pressures. It is worth finding ways of documenting effectiveness and also cultivating sources of support in advance.
- Services can experience pressure as a result of failing to meet their aims of utilising community resources, or placing service users in other settings: in setting up the service it is important to be modest about what can be achieved, especially in the early days.

Examples from Manchester

Within Manchester day services, as a whole, are still directly managed by the social services department. However, the Joint Service has developed a number of initiatives which, whilst not in themselves necessarily unique, arise in response to conditions 'on the ground' and contain innovative features.

The Northfield Project

One day centre in North Manchester accommodated a high proportion of people with multiple physical disabilities. This brought into focus a dissatisfaction with the effectiveness of the model of additional health support provided by individual practitioners going into day services on an ad hoc basis.

In October 1993 Northfield Special Needs Unit was established, following the closure of a large traditional adult training centre.. This unit initially had 21 service users, of whom 70 per cent used wheelchairs. The project was established with a management committee made up of the day centre manager, the team manager from the community learning disability team and a physiotherapist from the community team.

In addition to the management team there were named health professionals (occupational therapy, physiotherapy, speech and language therapy, psychology and community nursing) who dedicated a minimum of four hours each week to the project.

Initial experience suggested that the management committee was an unwieldy and unresponsive tool for resolving day-to-day service problems. It was therefore supplemented by the creation of the post of clinical coordinator, a health practitioner who, at this stage, dedicated a minimum of 16 hours each week to the project. This person also managed a health support worker, employed for 20 hours a week to work alongside practitioners developing a detailed knowledge of service users' programmes and the delivery of support, knowledge and skills which were shared with day centre officers. Many service users had difficulty with feeding and, in response to this, two lunchtime support workers were employed to offer very targeted and focused extra support (a model which has since been taken up by other day services in the city).

The clinical coordinator also jointly chaired the 'quality action group' consisting of parents, carers, day centre officers, the unit manager and independent members, which met every two months to address issues of service delivery.

The health staff working on the project advised on modifications to the building's structure and the purchase of new equipment/aids so that both were driven by established service user need. In turn, health practitioners have gained a more thorough understanding of the service needs as a whole than would have been possible under traditional working arrangements. An example is the improved risk management of problems with swallowing which has resulted in a reduction in respiratory problems. Care plans are carried through with a greater consistency than before. Staff training needs have been identified and tackled by means of small group training and skill-sharing in the workplace.

Perhaps the most marked changes have been in areas which are more difficult to measure – in the atmosphere, the openness and sense of common purpose between workers from different disciplines and different agencies. Staff who work full-time within a setting can resent health practitioners, perceiving them as heaping extra requirements on an already stretched situation which they don't understand. The Northfield Project, with its structure of attached health professionals and health support workers, has led to a more positive approach across agencies. Roles seem to be mutually understood and a good grasp of the rationale behind programmes, as well as the details of prescribed practice, is evident.

Recently, the established nature and effective operation of the service systems has enabled the clinical coordinator role to change to that of 'clinical adviser' – a semantic shift which reflects a stepping back from day-to-day involvement.

Small-scale pilot projects are markedly vulnerable to staff turnover. The Northfield Special Care Unit has been hit particularly hard, as the community learning disability teams were restructured some 18 months after the project began and only two members of the original health team maintained an involvement. At the same time there was a more than 50 per cent turnover in the complement of day centre officers. The overall success of the unit owes much to the commitment of those with a continuing involvement. It reinforces the general principle that, given the possibility of staff change, it is effective structures and clear, detailed aims and objectives that safeguard quality.

Drop-ins

Until recently, the Joint Service's only other involvement in daytime provision had been the development of 'drop-ins' which developed as it became increasingly obvious that large numbers of people within the Joint Service's staffed residential provision received no day-service whatsoever. Other people who received no daytime support were those living in residential settings staffed by the private and voluntary sectors, as well as people living independently with minimal support.

At their most basic, drop-ins offered 'somewhere to go, something to do and some people to meet' and did so without the necessity (by and large) of finding additional resources. The first drop-ins were organised by members of fieldwork teams with those attending often bringing residential staff with them, and occasional sessional workers also having some input. One of the first drop-ins, for example, made use of an art therapist on a sessional basis. The activities on offer included arts and crafts, music, sports activities, recreational games and the opportunity for social contact.

There have also been attempts to offer drop-ins on a slightly different basis. A reduction in service offered by a local adult training centre left nine individuals with special needs with only two days each week at their day service. A drop-in was suggested as a possible response to this. The nine people in question were perceived to be quite challenging, and the loose social nature of the established drop-ins was perceived as not meeting their needs. A more structured format was produced, making greater use of sessional workers in art therapy, music and drama and aromatherapy.

More definitive and structured programmes have also been attempted within the looser framework of the original drop-ins; a mixed group of 12 people met regularly to work on the Patterns for Living course, while another group worked on issues of sexuality and relationships.

A service for people with autism

The Joint Service also manages and partly staffs a complex needs day service. The roots of this project go back to a specialist drop-in which was operated for two days a week over several months in 1992. It was specifically targeted at people with relatively complex needs, often with autism or autistic characteristics, who had recently been resettled from two of the hostels and was led by an occupational therapist who coordinated the activity of direct care staff who supported those who attended. The project was set up in a room within a community centre in Fallowfield, and ran in the mornings for three days per week. The project established the value of a structured approach, resulting in high levels of purposeful behaviour in a variety of largely developmental and educational activities. It was seen as a good example of how NHS professional leadership can enable direct care staff to work effectively with 'hard to serve' service users.

At the same time, the model of 'clinically managed social care' (see Chapter 12) had been developed to improve provision to people with severe behavioural problems.

On the basis of these positive experiences, the new Joint Service was approached, in 1994, to help resolve a problem in serving one autistic young man who attended one of the day services. His behaviour had become difficult to manage within that setting and, despite efforts to resolve this through joint work with specialist staff in the community team based at the centre, his placement had broken down. One option was to recruit staff to provide an individual service which would have been very costly and probably claustrophobic both for the service user and the staff. Instead, it was suggested that the social services department switch some of its resources to create a small service catering for up to six young adults with autistic characteristics who were being poorly served within the existing provision.

The project was established in late August 1994 to offer daytime activities for ultimately five or six people with complex needs relating to autism. It is managed by a nurse employed by the Mancunian Trust as project leader and staffed by two day centre officers, drawn from existing day services, who are managed and supervised by the project leader but remain employed by social services. In addition there is a part-time unqualified member of staff employed for 16 hours a week by the Trust.

The project leader is managed by, and receives clinical supervision from, the Joint Service's head of development and clinical services (who is also a clinical psychologist) and maintains professional links through the Trust's practice advisers for nursing.

The service is delivered from rooms adjoining a social services day centre. At first sight it resembles a special care section rather more radically separate from the mainstream provision than is generally regarded as good practice (this issue of integration will be returned to later). In the original service specification it was agreed that the fabric of the building would remain the responsibility of the day centre manager. Work on risk assessment indicated the need for extensive and expensive modifications – for example, the use of polycarbonate windows.

The approach used by the project is eclectic. Considerable use is made of ideas and methods derived from the North American TEACCH programme (Mesibov *et al.*, 1994). Service users are taught, and helped to use, a visual planning display, both for structure and predictability across the day and (less frequently) for individual activities, in order to reduce the levels of anxiety experienced in 'looser' social situations.

The spread of activities contained within this structure can broadly be divided into: the development of educational and social skills, including detailed communication programmes; the development of self-help; leisure and recreational skills; and activities derived from the work of Geoffrey Waldon (see Waldon, 1985).

Since it was believed that anxiety experienced by service users had been the root cause of the sorts of behavioural challenges which they had presented in other environments, it was envisaged that this anxiety would be reduced by a predictable, structured day that offered understandable, purposeful activity, in an environment much less crowded, noisy and chaotic than found in most day services. The emphasis on skills development would also offer people alternative and more constructive means to meet their needs (Donnellan *et al.*, 1988). It was also felt that staff who could focus on understanding the difficulties faced by people with autism would be in a better position to support them.

In recognition of the fact that behavioural challenges were unlikely to simply vanish, applied behaviour analysis seemed to offer the best available means to understand the causation of particular behaviours. Thus regular and detailed records of behaviour are made on a daily basis for all service users, in addition to records of specific incidents. This has provided staff with a detailed working knowledge of setting factors, precursors, triggers and cycles of escalation for what are often quite complexly determined behaviours.

Multidisciplinary input to the project has also been vital, with psychology, speech and language therapy, occupational therapy and nursing all making contributions to assessment and the devising of positive programmes. Again, behavioural recording and multidisciplinary assessment formed part of the initial service specification and are built into the monitoring of the project.

The service also tackles the issue of social integration through the increased use of community resources. Re-entry to mainstream day services is not seen as a particularly pertinent goal, given the past history of the majority of service users. This does mean that the project remains isolated and has created problems in terms of covering for sickness (which is fortunately very low, running at around 3 per cent) and in terms of 'succession' should a member of staff leave the project.

As with the clinically managed houses (see Chapter 12), a structure of regular, fortnightly service user reviews, fortnightly staff meetings and team review days (three per year) enables the coordination of the team's work and the monitoring of progress towards service user goals. This framework complements and informs regular individual supervision of staff as well as the monitoring of the overall service via an audit of quality standards.

Similarly, the structure of post-incident debriefing is also being reviewed to facilitate the offer of emotional support whilst encouraging reflective practice by means of an examination of the causes of an incident and the effectiveness and practicality of current interventions.

Initially, the project offered daytime support to only one service user – the young man in his mid-twenties who lived in the family home (mentioned above). He was joined, within a few months, by two more – a young woman who had recently left school and for whom it was proving difficult to provide a service, and a second woman who was inappropriately placed in an existing day centre which she had attended for some considerable time, as demonstrated by the radical degree of withdrawal she displayed in that setting.

By July 1995 considerable and demonstrable progress had been made in the areas of engagement in a range of activities (including increasing use of ordinary community facilities) and in lessening the frequency and severity of behavioural crises. At this point, a fourth service user joined the group which has remained constant up to the present.

By October 1995 it had become clear that there was a serious incompatibility between the most newly introduced member and an existing service user. This could not have been anticipated and necessitated a long period of reactive crisis management. In effect the two service users received separate, but parallel, services which have been highly intensive of staff time and effectively delayed entry of a fifth person until the time of writing. The service has been maintained for both men and targets, in terms of reductions in intensity of support, increase in purposeful engagement and reductions in inappropriate behaviours, have been met for all service users.

Small-scale projects are vulnerable to problems of this sort and both provider managers and purchasers must have some understanding of the nature of the difficulties entailed (as they did in this case). Fortunately, the service specification had built in the possibility of forestalling the introduction of new service users at crisis points, and also contains exit criteria.

External monitoring by the social services purchasing team has been comprehensive and detailed. There has been a recognition of need and satisfaction with the service provided. Negotiations have begun on commissioning a second site for the service. This development would go a considerable way towards solving the problem of service user incompatibility and reduce the problems of the vulnerability of such a small staff pool to sickness or staff movement.

The complex needs day service recognises that some people need carefully designed specialised supports. The service uses both specialised (currently segregated) settings and local community resources. The provision is for people who have displayed extreme behavioural challenges in the past, and may still do so in the present and foreseeable future. The service therefore represents a compromise between specialist skilled input and setting design, and access to ordinary settings, people and identity-conferring activities.

Jobs through LETS

In contrast to the above developments, the Joint Service is exploring novel ways of helping the community more fully include its learning-disabled members through alternative forms of economic activity and community development.

LETS stands for Local Exchange Trading Scheme. Originally developed in Canada, there are now over 500 such schemes in the UK. They enable members of a community to exchange services and goods, independently from the formal monetary economy, on the basis of an exchange of a notional currency. In Manchester this is the 'bobbin'. So one person cleans another person's upstairs windows and is paid in bobbins. He spends the bobbins on a lift to the next city. The person who drives him uses the bobbins for someone to sit with her elderly mother and so on. The system encourages the creation of social networks, as well as making goods and services available that would otherwise require money: at its best, a LETS builds a community and creates real wealth. As such, it has interesting possibilities for learning-disabled people and their allies, offering them opportunity to use their skills to provide services people want and to make contact with members of the local community whom they might not otherwise meet. It also offers participation in economic activity without the problem of the benefit trap.

Recently, learning-disabled people in Manchester have begun to participate in the local LETS. So far six people are involved in one part of the city. They have worked on a monthly recycling round, on collecting paper and glass to be recycled, on leafleting, on packaging food and done office work. This has been a positive experience for the people concerned, but also presents some dilemmas and problems to work on.

Some people need support to participate in the activities of the LETS, and the presence of a staff member can be a barrier. The LETS scheme itself is being explored as a source of this support.

Access to an informal network is valuable but, for the service, a dilemma arises concerning whether people need to be vetted (as for a volunteer scheme, for example). This probably depends on the activity involved. For example, one person was offered an excursion by car in exchange for 'bobbins' he had earned. This would be no problem for someone who could reasonably make a judgement about the risk involved in this arrangement but, in this situation, staff had to decide for the person. There is clearly a balance to be struck between protecting vulnerable people and encouraging participation in networks: we have learned more about the importance of both these things in recent years.

Conclusion

The chapter began with reference to *Better Services for the Mentally Handicapped* a White Paper published in 1971. It recognised that the hospital closure programme would necessitate an attendant growth in opportunities in the community for daytime occupation.

There has been a growth in employment services and adult education courses for learning-disabled people. Financial constraints have led organisations providing these services to concentrate on outcomes; admission is now determined on a judgement that a trainee or student can move on to the next stage. The chapter has also explored the shortfall of the 'readiness model' for the most disabled people in the community.

An attempt also has been made to describe what a good quality day care service would look like and what skills and experience would be required of staff. The chapter reviewed the need to access the local community and how this would impact on where a service might be based. It also identified the internal and external pressure of providing a day service and explored the benefits of specialisation.

References and resources

Allen, D. (1994), 'Towards meaningful daytime activity' in E. Emerson, P. McGill and J. Mansell (eds), *Severe Learning Disabilities and Challenging Behaviours: Designing High Quality Services*, London: Chapman and Hall.

Barnes, H., North, P. and Walker, P. (1996), *LETS on Low Income*, London: New Economics Foundation.

Department of Health and Social Security (1971), *Better Services for the Mentally Handicapped*, London: HMSO.

Donnellan, A.M., La Vigna, G.W., Negri-Shoultz, N. and Fassbender, L.L. (1988), *Progress Without Punishment*, New York: Teachers College Press.

Lang, P. (1994), *LETS Work: Rebuilding the Local Economy*, London: Grover Books.

Mesibov, G.B., Schopler, E. and Hearsey, K.A. (1994), 'Structured teaching' in E. Schopler and G.B. Mesibov (eds), *Behavioural Issues in Autism*, New York: Plenum.

National Development Group (1977), *Pamphlet No. 5: Day Services for Mentally Handicapped Adults*, London: HMSO.

Richards, V. (1983), *Why Work?*, London: Freedom Press.

Waldon, G. (1985), *Understanding Understanding*, Manchester: The Centre for Learning to Learn More Effectively.

9 Developing and managing therapy practice

Jane Jolliffe, Sylvia Jones, Lynsay Juffs,
Cathi McKessy, Linda Prinsloo, Rachel Samuels,
Moira Speechley and Debbie Windley
with contributions by Mark Burton

Introduction

For the purposes of this chapter, the 'therapy professions' are speech and language therapy, occupational therapy and physiotherapy. Sometimes erroneously referred to as PAMS (professions ancillary to medicine) they are in fact distinctive disciplines, each with its own body of knowledge and practice. Nationally, it seems that there has been some neglect of this aspect of community learning disability services, with few staff, often professionally isolated and poorly integrated into service provision. The emphasis in provision has been on the larger staff groups of nurses and social workers/ care managers while, in terms of promotion of novel approaches to practice, it has been the small, but vocal, psychology profession that has made much of the running.

This chapter briefly reviews some of the issues in organising the therapy professions in community learning disability services, and then offers a 'showcase' for some of the leading-edge practice developed in recent years in the Manchester Joint Service.

Key issues

Professional leadership and service management

Chapters 2 and 3 on designing the organisation and leading and supporting staff respectively, review issues in providing structures that give both adequate accountability and sufficient professional guidance and support. Essentially, there are two options for organising these staff:

1 separate department(s), either of therapy services, or of each separate therapy profession
2 integration of the staff into the interdisciplinary teams.

If option 1 is adopted, then a separate referral system is required, as well as some means for ensuring that these staff share the same priorities as the rest of the service. There is also the question of whether management should be provided by the learning disability service or by the therapy department of the wider organisation. Our own experience is that there is a great advantage in the learning disability service managing all the interdisciplinary components. Fragmentation, professional rivalry and poor accountability for resource use can result from situations where a generic department (or, worse, another organisation) provides one of the elements.

If option 2 is adopted, then there needs to be effective arrangements for professional supervision and leadership. Otherwise, staff will feel isolated and risk losing touch with developments in knowledge and practice in their discipline. The model of practice advisers and professional supervision set out in the Appendix gives one way of meeting this requirement. If this requirement is met, then the interaction among the disciplines in the interdisciplinary (not merely multidisciplinary) team is itself a rich source of innovative strategies. It is also important that the heads of the professions outside the learning disability service understand the arrangements and continue to give professional support where required.

Recruitment

The NHS has failed to train and retain sufficient therapy professionals. Moreover, for reasons that remain obscure, work with learning-disabled people appears to be unattractive to many therapists. At the time of writing, recruitment difficulties are most severe in physiotherapy; market forces, as ever, are distorting and weakening social provision, with physiotherapists being able to command higher salaries in the private sector, such as sports injury clinics, or in the USA.

Speech and language therapy also faces recruitment difficulties. Although, as yet, these are less severe, the high level of need for speech and language therapy among learning-disabled people does mean that these staff are under considerable referral pressure (see below).

Recruitment difficulties are likely to remain for some time, but can be ameliorated with the following strategies:

- **Develop a critical mass of staff**. It is difficult to recruit into a weak and overloaded service.
- **Legitimate mutual support among staff in a discipline**. This is most useful if linked to the professional support system and underpinned by a commitment to high standards.
- **Establish a 'name'**. This can be done locally, regionally, and nationally – for example, through sharing developments in practice.
- **Encourage both continued education and training of therapy staff**. This should be combined with the creation of opportunities for them to train other workers.
- **Maintain contact with colleagues in other specialities**. These might include paediatric special needs and mental health.

Balancing proactive and reactive work

Pressure of referrals means that careful prioritisation is required. This will ensure those most in need (for example, for speech and language therapists, those with eating and swallowing difficulties and those with communication-related behavioural problems) are seen and ensures that therapists can share their knowledge and skills with other staff. There is a balance to be struck here: because a scarce resource cannot provide for everyone, indirect work via others can be more productive, as long as care is taken to ensure that the knowledge and skills disseminated are not so diluted or distorted as to be ineffective, or worse, dangerous. It is also demoralising if the job merely involves labouring away at a long waiting list that is added to as quickly as people are seen. On the other hand, time spent in development and training is time that could otherwise be used in individual work. Groundrules should therefore be established and agreed, based on an understanding of the likely outcomes of individual assessment and intervention, indirect work via other staff, and through service development.

Practice developments in Manchester

It is difficult to develop and manage a service without an understanding of its practice base. This section illustrates the variety of contributions made by therapy staff to the work of the service.

What follows is a selective review of work done by speech and language therapists and occupational therapists in the Manchester Joint Service. The recruitment difficulties discussed above have meant that, although innovative work has been carried out in the past, physiotherapists have recently been largely concerned to meet basic requirements for care, albeit of a high standard (Maitland *et al.*, 1996; Lally, *et al.*, 1995a, 1995b). As in the similar case of clinical psychology, recruitment problems are being tackled by the development of a career structure for unqualified assistants, with varying degrees of experience and training, who work under the supervision of qualified staff.

Speech and language therapy developments

Eating, drinking and swallowing guidelines

An increasing number of referrals for eating, drinking and swallowing assessments for adults created a need for the speech and language therapists to develop written guidance for parents and carers assisting the individual person to eat and drink. These eating and drinking guidelines are now established and implemented at the completion of the individual's assessment and are used in all the learning disability teams. Reflecting the multidisciplinary nature of the support required by people with dysphagia, they draw together information from various sources including the individual, their carers, the speech and language therapist, dietician, physiotherapist and medical staff. The guidelines are as follows:

- Be aware of the risks to the person during eating and drinking after they have been identified by the speech and language therapist at assessment.
- Understand the risks to the person in order to minimise them.
- Have clear and accessible guidelines to follow when assisting the person to eat and drink to encourage consistency and good practice.
- Have a list of people to contact (for example, GP, speech and language therapist, physiotherapist, dietician). This provides easy reference should any difficulties arise, more training is required on further investigations or advice are needed.
- Provide a comprehensive record of the person's eating and drinking difficulties to be updated as necessary. Full written information is important for new carers who may be assisting the person to eat, as well as training and having discussions with the existing care staff and speech and language therapist involved.
- Encourage a small, consistent group of carers to provide assistance at the person's mealtimes, and ask them to read and sign that they have understood the guidelines.
- Provide a summary of the guidelines' main points to put in an easily

visible place (for example, inside a kitchen cupboard door) to remind carers.

How were the guidelines drawn up? Speech and language therapists in the Joint Service hold regular quality circle meetings in which issues and developments related to working practice are discussed, reviewed and introduced. When considering drawing up the guidelines we reviewed existing formats used by colleagues in paediatric and adult hospital-based services. We incorporated information which we considered to be important for learning-disabled adults and their support services. A format was drawn up with main headings as a guide to completion for each person.

The drafted guidelines were then commented on and trialled in practice to highlight any further additional headings which were required to include all information relevant in a clear and comprehensive way. A final format was agreed and has been in operation since 1996.

What do the guidelines involve? The eating, drinking and swallowing guidelines include the following headings:

- *Title page.* This includes the name of the person and the date of the guidelines.
- *List of contacts.* This includes, for example, GP, speech and language therapist, physiotherapist, community nurse, dietician.
- *Background information.* This includes the reason for referral, particular concerns and relevant medical information.
- *What is the problem?* This section details the difficulties which the person experiences with eating, drinking and swallowing and the potential risks to them – for example, the risks of aspiration (taking food or fluid into the lungs), asphyxiation and the risks of not obtaining enough food and fluid.
- *Positioning.* This details how the person should be positioned during eating and drinking to minimise risks of aspiration and to maximise opportunities for communication and achieving rapport during meals. Guidelines can also include more detailed seating information, drawn up by the physiotherapist involved, which may include pictures and a photograph and advice for the person assisting at mealtimes to protect their own back from strain and injury.
- *Equipment:* This section lists the equipment recommended by the speech and language therapist and occupational therapist to enable the person to take food and drink safely. The guidelines may also include a list of suppliers of the equipment and details of who can obtain them.

- *Consistency of food.* Here, the safest food consistency is described and examples of food of this consistency are given – for example, a soft, thick, smooth consistency with no lumps, bits or pieces of food in it, such as smooth thick mashed potato. Further description and examples of foods of the consistency required can be added in the appendices.
- *Foods to avoid*: This details foods, textures and consistencies that are unsafe for the person.
- *Drinks to avoid.* This details the consistency of drinks that are unsafe for the person.
- *What to do when giving the person something to eat.* This section details the procedure – including position, equipment, communication, food consistency and pacing – in order for the person to eat as safely as possible and with respect and comfort.
- *What to do when giving the person a drink.* This details the procedure as above but for drinking.
- *Food and drink likes and dislikes.* Here the person's favourite and least favourite foods and drinks are detailed.
- *Any special requirements.* This section records any dietary requirements, including food intolerances and religious requirements.
- *Signatures.* Here, the carers and parents, who have read, understood and had the opportunity to discuss the guidelines with the speech and language therapist, sign to show this.
- *Summary page.* Here, the key points of the guidelines are listed in a 'dos and don'ts' format to be pulled out and placed in an easily readable position.

The information included in the guidelines has proved invaluable as a training tool, providing comprehensive information which can be reviewed as appropriate and guiding good practice. The guidelines can be included in an individual 'care package' to ensure that they are implemented in all settings that the person uses, and can be audited in the future.

Eating and drinking questionnaire

While working with our increasing caseload of adults with eating, drinking and swallowing difficulties, it became clear that carers often omitted important background information, usually because they thought it 'irrelevant'. What was needed was a clear way of collecting necessary information from all concerned. Contacting all sources, including other professionals and the GP as well as the carers of the person, revealed more information than talking to one set of carers alone.

The eating and drinking questionnaire was devised at the quality circle meetings to guide written collation of all the relevant information. It is intended to be discussed and completed with all carers and service users before an observational assessment is carried out.

The questionnaire was designed to:

- collate information on the person's medical background information
- find out current practices for assisting the person to eat and drink – for example, the consistency of food and drink usually given and the equipment and position used – and who is involved
- collect other information relevant to an eating and drinking assessment and subsequent guidelines – for example, client's weight, episodes of vomiting, dental status and health, hearing and vision, past medical conditions which may not immediately be connected with swallowing difficulties (for instance, hiatus hernia, anaemia, dehydration)
- allow carers and parents to make a note of their concerns when assisting the person
- find out the person's likes and dislikes in terms of food and drink and any special dietary requirements
- ask carers and parents how they think the person is managing food and drink in their mouths – for example, whether food or drink ever comes down the person's nose, whether the person can chew foods and whether gagging or coughing occurs during mealtimes.
- find out whether the person has regular chest care or chest infections
- establish the training needs of the carers assisting the person to eat and drink and any relevant training which they may have already received, including resuscitation and attendance on the locally run course 'Introduction to eating, drinking and swallowing problems'.

The questionnaire has proved a valuable tool for collecting information to guide assessment and future input.

The risk management plan

Within the service, risk assessments and risk management plans had been devised or drawn up in situations where risk needed to be quantified and managed or reduced – for example, where service users live independently or access community facilities without support. As the issue of supporting service users with eating and drinking difficulties within a day centre setting became paramount, the same model was applied.

The risk management plan was drawn up initially in consultation with social services day centre officers and speech and language therapists expe-

Table 9.1 Example chart for risk 1: asphyxiation

Method[1]	Feasibility[2]	Likely effectiveness[3]	Appropriateness[4]	Actions/conclusions[5]
Offer food of an appropriate consistency – for example, mashed or liquidised.	High.	Likely to considerably reduce risk but 100 per cent reduction cannot be guaranteed.	Appropriate. Slight restriction to the range of foods experienced is offset by the gains in safety	1. Initiate investigations by specialists to determine the appropriate consistency. 2. Discuss definition of consistency with kitchen and care staff. Liaise with kitchen staff to ensure that food is prepared to the appropriate consistency. 3. Review budget for special dietary needs and equipment. etc ...

Notes:
1 Suggests ways of reducing or alleviating the risk.
2 Indicates how practical the method would be to implement.
3 Indicates how suitable the method could be for the person.
4 Makes a judgement about how far the risk could be reduced or prevented by employing the method chosen.
5 Lists agreed action and any requirements needed to carry out the method.

rienced in supporting people with eating and drinking difficulties. After subsequent drafts were completed, further consultation with physiotherapists, dieticians and community nurses was carried out. Around this time the document was piloted with a number of service users accessing day services and residential services so that its usefulness, in helping support workers identify risks and work towards reducing or alleviating those risks or consequences, could be assessed.

For each risk the following headings are used:

- Method
- Feasibility
- Appropriateness
- Likely effectiveness
- Actions and conclusions.

These are presented in chart form as illustrated in Table 9.1.

The risk management plan is usually completed by the speech and language therapist and the support workers or carer. Agreement is reached regarding the risks which the person may be facing and the actions needed to alleviate these. The relevant sections are highlighted along with the actions. The document is then kept with the person's records after being signed by those who completed the plan and agreed the actions. Managers, as well as direct carers, should be involved to highlight the shared responsibility and the necessity of action from managers regarding, for example, adequate cover, training provision, additional budgets for dietary changes and so on.

Once completed, the actions agreed in the risk management plan are used when drawing up guidelines. In using the plan this way it has been found that carers and support workers are able to appreciate the risks and necessary actions to be carried out. Joint ownership is also achieved. In addition, if a person's skills deteriorate, the plan provides a useful framework for re-evaluation. Carers and support workers can see clearly the revised actions that are necessary by referring to the plan. If all the actions have been previously implemented without the risks being reduced as desired, the issue of medical or surgical interventions can be raised as a natural progression.

Future plans and developments relating to dysphagia management

Since the formation of the Joint Learning Disability Service, the dysphagia service offered by the speech and language therapists has evolved dramatically. Assessment and management have been standardised across the city, along with the writing of appropriate policy documents outlining the elements of the service. A further development has been the introduction of the two-day in-service training course for carers. A two-hour 'roadshow' is being piloted to raise awareness amongst staff who would not feel it appropriate to attend the two-day course.

An audit, to be carried out with the clinical audit department, is also being conducted for people discharged or on review. Its aim is to establish:

- the presence and use of specified utensils
- the presence and use of the guidelines
- the training received by the current support workers and carers.

The interest in dysphagia management by the senior managers of the service is further indicated by their commitment to developing the risk management plan into an effective tool for use not only within Manchester but further afield. The plan is likely to be published in the near future.

Communication assessment with people exhibiting behavioural challenges

As other chapters demonstrate, many learning-disabled people do present behavioural challenges at some point in their lives. It has been found that there is an association between challenging behaviour and unmet individual need (see, for example, Kiernan and Qureshi, 1993; DoH, 1993). A local survey (Speake and Kellaway, 1992) found that 31 per cent of service users had no verbal communication, while figures of between 50 and 89 per cent have been reported as the proportion with some kind of communication difficulty (Van der Gaag and Dormandy, 1993). These severe communication difficulties lead to considerable difficulties in recognising the individual needs of many learning-disabled people, which could contribute significantly to the problem of challenging behaviour. Speech and language therapists are having to adapt their skills to this issue.

There has been a widespread use of the 'communicative hypothesis' concerning the function of much challenging behaviour (Carr and Durand, 1985), which suggests that behavioural challenges occur because the person is unable to express their needs and wants through verbal means and therefore substitutes highly noticeable behaviours as a means of eliciting support, changing stimulation levels, terminating or initiating an activity and so on.

Other disciplines (especially psychology) have made a contribution to this work (Durand, 1990; Carr *et al.*, 1993) but, although it is rooted in behavioural psychology, this work has not been informed by a contemporary systematic analysis of communication (cf. Calculator and Bedrossian, 1988; Kiernan *et al.*, 1987).

From our own clinical practice and analysis of the literature we have developed a second communicative hypothesis, that:

> ... challenging behaviour may occur when communication towards the person with a learning disability does not match their receptive communicative competence (capacity to understand).

We find that a significant proportion of problem behaviours take place when care givers do not communicate in ways that the learning-disabled person can understand: as a result, communication and the verbal environment is likely to be experienced as confusing, anxiety-arousing, overwhelming and/or threatening.

Taking both the original communicative hypothesis and our second hypothesis together, we can suggest that a great deal of challenging behaviour occurs as a consequence of a mismatch between the communicative competence of the learning-disabled person and the strategies used to communicate with that person and to mediate environmental events. This mirrors the analysis of social skill as the joint competence of individual and social setting (Burton and Kagan, 1995).

In the absence of a strong body of research, we can provide illustrations from our work (see the 'Examples' overleaf).

We have drawn on current understanding of syntactic, semantic and pragmatic aspects of communication (for example, Peccei, 1994; Van der Gaag and Dormandy, 1993; Van der Gaag, 1988) to develop a rigorous assessment schedule (Jolliffe, 1996). This yields practical guidance to care givers on appropriate ways of communicating with the person who may exhibit challenging behaviour – for example, by using photographs, object cue systems, or altering the vocabulary and syntax used in speech. This communicative analysis also provides a basis for building on the person's precommunicative and communicative repertoire, enabling important wants and needs to be recognised. Intervention is carried out with individual service users, usually by working through their staff teams. To date, most work has been via client-specific staff training workshops which cover general issues, and through clinical consultation with direct care staff and their supervisors, utilising written communication guidelines based on the assessment. This seems to represent an efficient use of the scarce speech and language therapy resource, but there is scope for the development of both the assessment and intervention methodologies, and for the rigorous evaluation of the deployment of speech and language therapists in this way.

Examples: communication-related challenging behaviours

1 A man with autism has a good vocabulary and speaks clearly. He has difficulties in decoding pragmatic aspects of communication, which lead him habitually to assume that conversations refer to him. Thus, when someone else is asked to make coffee he also attempts to carry out the task, entering into conflict with staff who have already asked him to do something different. He is confused when asked to return to his seat because, as far as he is concerned, he has just been asked to get up and make coffee.

2 A woman understands the word 'no', but does not interpret utterances involving 'not' (or 'n't') as negatives. As a result, she frequently has the experience of being told (as far as she is concerned) that something is going to happen and then becoming frustrated when it does not.

3 A woman uses the word 'Coke' to mean any cold drink. She asks for 'Coke', receives it and throws it on the floor.

4 A man has a varied life in the community, having been resettled from a mental handicap hospital. On one outing by rail he expects a train to stop but it goes on through the station. Staff have no way of explaining that this is not the train they are waiting for, and he hits one of them.

5 A man with severe learning disability has a small vocabulary and can understand simple utterances. When people direct more complex utterances at him he becomes highly stressed, striking out and hitting his head.

Note:
Although the above vignettes involve some speculation, the interpretations are consistent with what is known about the communicative abilities of the people concerned, and similar sequences of events have been noted on several occasions for each person.

Assessment work can be informed by literature now emerging on the communication and language development of people with various developmental disabilities (for example, Paul, *et al.*, 1987; Tager-Flusberg, 1989; Tager-Flusberg *et al.*, 1990), as well as the language development of non-disabled people (for example, Peccei, 1994).

A research proposal to progress this work has been developed with colleagues at Manchester Metropolitan University.

Occupational therapy developments

Sensory integration

Sensory integration (SI) is an approach which analyses a person's ability to cope with sensory information and make sense of it, by focusing on their response to vestibular, proprioceptive, and tactile stimuli. Underresponsiveness or overresponsiveness to these stimuli will affect the person's behaviour and ability to learn.

We are all constantly making unconscious decisions about which sensations we take notice of, and are therefore modulating our response. For example, when watching television we may focus on what we are seeing and hearing and ignore the feel of the chair or the clothes we are wearing, although we may automatically react to these by changing position. Someone with an SI problem may not filter sensory information properly, so the clothes feel unbearably tickly and the chair painfully hard. This may then explain why this person refuses to sit on a chair for any length of time and why they tear off their clothes: they would be significantly distracted from the television. For people with intellectual disabilities such difficulties could present as behavioural challenges and their reduced concentration could diminish opportunities for learning.

After reviewing the literature and attending courses on sensory integration, occupational therapists in the Joint Service decided to pilot the use of SI locally. We were excited by the opportunities which this approach offered to facilitate learning and behavioural change with some service users. Although SI has been primarily used within a paediatric setting with children with developmental dyspraxia and poor motor coordination, work has been done more recently with severely learning-disabled adults, the results of which appear promising.

Therapeutic application The aim of SI therapy is to introduce sensory stimuli in such a way as to improve the person's ability to modulate their response. This may involve the use of stimuli, which raise and lower arousal levels, being used simultaneously in order to bring about an optimum level of arousal and thus an ability to interact with the environment. An example might be being pushed on a swing (raising arousal levels) while surrounded by heavy cushions (lowering arousal levels). This has to be carried out in an environment where the person feels safe and in control.

As we learn more about the person's response to stimuli in individual sessions we are then able to make recommendations which can be implemented in the person's home or daytime environment. Similarly, recommendations can be made about how to bring about the optimal arousal levels before and after an activity, or about which activities are appropriate, or about the environment or clothing and so on.

Examples: application of SI therapy

1   One person benefited from having a heavy quilt wrapped around her when travelling by bus or car. From an SI perspective it would appear that the heavy pressure reduced the high arousal levels due to the vestibular stimulation from movement.

2   Another person was often agitated at bedtime and would refuse to go to bed, often staying up until the early hours, which was very difficult for his family. By introducing tactile stimulation – in this case light brushing to his palms and arms – his arousal levels were brought to a point where he was able to relax; this improved his tolerance to lying down in bed.

3   In a day service setting, we have worked at altering the environment and provided specific sensory input in order to increase a person's tolerance to social interaction and the opportunities this then offers to learn new skills. A 'den' area was created to enable her to feel more secure, and vestibular stimulation was introduced within this in order to raise her arousal levels and willingness to interact.

A pilot research study   An initial study is being undertaken to evaluate the usefulness of the SI approach. It involves people who demonstrate high or low arousal levels not currently explained by any other model and who exhibit poor motor coordination and/or tactile sensitivity. People with additional sensory impairments or significant physical disabilities are excluded from the pilot as the therapists themselves develop skills in identifying where SI dysfunction exists.

Initial screening was carried out by means of a lifestyle assessment derived from the *Sensory Integration Inventory for Adults with Developmental Disabilities* (Reisman and Hanschu, 1992). If this suggested a SI dysfunction, an in-depth assessment of response to vestibular, tactile and proprioceptive stimuli was conducted using clinical observations based on the assessment in the *MOTTO Sensory Approach* (Soper and Robinson-Thorley, 1995).

Therapeutic work based on the results of the assessment then takes place on a regular basis. Psychologist colleagues are helping with the complex task of evaluating changes resulting from the interventions.

Aromatherapy and massage

Aromatherapy and massage have been used for some time in Manchester, as elsewhere, with adult users of learning disability services. As with any treatment there is a danger that it will be applied inappropriately. Recently a protocol has been drawn up to ensure standards of practice and to enable the proper development of these therapeutic activities.

Who carries out treatment? Currently there is one occupational therapist who has the relevant qualifications in aromatherapy and massage, and two physiotherapists who are qualified in massage. Due to other professional commitments, ways of working have been established in order to meet the needs of those service users who might make use of these therapies.

Training in the techniques of hand and foot massage is given to staff working with an individual service user or group of service users, who have been identified as potentially benefiting from aromatherapy and massage. Treatment sessions can then be carried out under the supervision of the qualified therapist.

Where appropriate, service users are referred to independent therapists on the same basis as other members of the public.

Where does treatment take place? Treatments may be given in day service settings, people's homes or at the therapist's own practice.

Why is treatment requested? The most common request is to help facilitate relaxation and reduce stress. Other reasons for referral include:

- to promote activity and alertness
- to stimulate sensory awareness
- to facilitate and encourage interaction and communication
- to promote tolerance to touch
- to relax and mobilise joints
- to provide a pleasurable activity
- to generally improve physical health
- to help provide pain relief

What is offered? The qualified therapists carry out assessments and draw treatment plans. In the case of aromatherapy, oils are blended for the individual person which can then be used by support staff who have received appropriate training. Progress is recorded, and the treatment plan is regularly reviewed.

Treatments are confined to hand and foot massage only, with or without the use of essential oils, unless it is part of the whole treatment plan for the person to receive more specialised treatment, as in the case of physiotherapy.

When is treatment given?   How often someone receives treatment will vary according to need. While the ideal for one person might be 10 to 20 minutes every day, for another it might only be once a month. Frequency of treatment is determined both by staff availability and finances, if the service user is paying privately for independent treatment. Programmes often involve some intense input initially, and can then be spaced out. It is usually possible to devise a programme that is both therapeutically beneficial to the service user and realistic for the staff to carry out.

The creative arts

Creative activities are proving valued and successful arenas of work for occupational therapists working in the Joint Service.

An art group

Example: a case study

Amongst other things Mr L had been referred to Occupational Therapy to access various activities. Mr L finds it difficult to express his feelings. He has always enjoyed working with crayons and paper and has a good appreciation of colour. It was thought that art would be a good medium in which to work.

Previously Mr L had tried art classes at his local college of adult education, but these had not provided appropriate levels of support.

Initially, an artist was found, who was happy to work with Mr L at home but, after discussion with the network manager, it was decided to set up a group in the community so more people could benefit and Mr L would have an activity away from home.

With the committed support of network staff, Mr L, a founder member of the group, has been able to attend throughout. He is producing work that is both satisfying to himself, and valued by the community, having already sold some pieces of work.

The art group has been running since April 1994. It is held on a Friday, with two sessions, one in the morning, and one in the afternoon, both lasting one and a half hours. The venue is a community centre attached to a local

Methodist church. A room is rented for the day and permanent storage space is provided.

The group is organised by occupational therapy staff, a professional artist who is employed on a sessional basis and a volunteer from the community. More recently, a service user representative from each session has been attending service reviews and participating in the general running of the group – for example, purchasing equipment, looking at possible venues for an exhibition.

The group is open to anyone but is mostly used by service users living in South and Central Manchester. For those people who require additional help, staff support is seen as essential. However, staff are careful to work in such a way that the work produced is done by the participants themselves and not by the staff. A small fee is charged which goes towards rent, materials and equipment, framing, project work, refreshments, parties and exhibitions.

Visitors to the group are welcomed and frequent visits are made by other community centre users, other artists and students, and those on school work experience.

Some of the benefits of these sessions include:

- involvement in a valued creative medium and pursuit
- exercise of choice regarding tasks, materials and colours
- making friendships and rekindling old ones, both within the group but also within the community centre more generally (one man met his aunt whom he had not seen for many years)
- celebration of seasonal and personal events
- use of the integrated setting – for example, the luncheon club and the coffee bar
- development of skills: artworks have been purchased, as well as used as the basis for Christmas cards and booklet covers
- development of a personal style: individuality and personality emerges in the work.
- development of independence: individual projects may take the person away from the group to explore and visit such venues as art galleries, museums and parks.

Therapy-based creative activities: another perspective   A need was identified in the Wythenshawe area to focus attention on the use of creative activities for adults with more profound and multiple learning disabilities. The specialist skills and enthusiasm of an artist/art therapy trainee, clinical psychologist, musician and two occupational therapists have been drawn together to provide the group activities. In each group, the facilitators act as guides, giving focus and support, but the route which the projects take is determined by the group members.

The group's work is best described as 'goal-free', exploring the release of creativity through non-judgemental exploration of creative activities.

Many service users have limited communication and limited scope for expressing their emotions. Creative activities encourage choice and provide scope for fun, individuality, spontaneity and self-expression. They offer space and time, where the goals and aims are set by the person who is doing the activity, thus enhancing self-confidence through achievement.

This is a closed group consisting of six people. Themed art activities, using a variety of media (clay, plaster, sand, paper and material collage), are designed to enhance group members' sensory awareness.

Music activities: a percussion group

Example: a case study

Miss K is a young woman who has a visual impairment and a limited vocabulary. She uses her own personal sounds to communicate and can also use a few Makaton signs. When Miss K first attended the music sessions she would withdraw and distance herself from the rest of the group. Gradually, through replicating her own body sounds with the use of a percussion instrument, Miss K was gently encouraged to join in the group activity. She soon became an active group member and her own individual and melodic sound could be heard in unison with her fellow group members.

This activity takes place at one of the social services day centres. In a similar way to the art group, occupational therapists work together with a professional musician, as well as day service staff. The musician is employed on a sessional basis, funded by the day service and the Joint Service. People with a wide variety of abilities attend for a two-hour session with a 15-minute teabreak which allows for socialisation.

The musician provides a wide variety of percussion instruments from different parts of the world. While some people explore these instruments independently, for others the emphasis is on the sensory experience of feeling the vibrations and listening to the different sounds from the various instruments.

Applications of microtechnology

What is microtechnology? Here the term 'microtechnology' is used to describe the computers and switching systems used to increase the control that multiple and profoundly disabled people have over their environments. Equipment consists of touch screen, keyboard, mouse, switches of various types and a variety of programs with specific outputs, such as visual and auditory feedback. The input devices and programs are chosen to match the specific needs and characteristics of the individual.

Switching systems have been introduced into various environments and consist of input devices – that is, a switch controlled by hand, elbow, head movement and so on – and the control box which is linked to output devices which can include most electrical equipment, including music systems, fans, and lights.

Why use microtechnology? When using switches or computers the reward is instant and consistent. The output must be of interest to the person using it in order to encourage its use and to establish the relationship between actions and effects.

Examples: microtechnology intervention

1 Peter has recently moved to supported housing, having previously lived in a large institution. He has quadraplegia. Due to his body shape, he has to sit in a reclining position at all times. He has no speech and indicates preferences by pointing to options presented to him. He is able to understand choices and the relationship between cause and effect. His support staff were keen that he had control over his environment. A switch system was introduced, initially to control his music system (his main interest) and special lighting in his bedroom. He then progressed to using the switch to control the food processor and microwave so that he can take part in preparing his meals. Peter will soon be using the switch to control a carousel projector, for recreational use, but also as a means of participating fully in meetings and reviews. Switch use has developed his ability to make choices, control activities and, we think, it has increased his self-esteem. It has expanded the range of opportunities available both to himself and the staff who support him. Peter is now perceived as a more active member of his household.

2 Tony attends a day centre where he has access to an Acorn computer. He has some difficulty coordinating his movements but is able to

---

control the computer by using gross motor movements directed towards the touch screen. The programs initially selected required random touching of the screen to elicit a response but, with practice, Tony has been able to direct his hand movements to a specific place on the screen to activate it. Tony enjoys these sessions, and is learning to anticipate, wait and plan his actions.

Microtechnology is advancing all the time, and the increased knowledge and confidence of therapy staff means that it can be made available to increase opportunity and control to people who would otherwise lack the means to influence their immediate environment.

Conclusion

This chapter has described some examples of the considerable contribution made by therapists working with learning-disabled people. It began with a description of the options for professional leadership and service management and argues the case for the integration of staff into interdisciplinary teams with effective arrangements for professional support and leadership.

The difficulties of recruitment and the pressure of referrals were described and some suggestions made of how to ameliorate the impact of these. The need to balance proactive and reactive work is explained.

There followed examples of innovative practice: guidelines for managing eating, drinking and swallowing disorders; communication assessment for people exhibiting behavioural challenges; the sensory integration project; aromatherapy and massage guidance; work in the creative arts and music; and microtechnology.

References and resources

Burton, M. and Kagan, C. (1995), *Social Skills for People with Learning Disabilities: A Social Capability Approach*, London: Chapman and Hall.

Calculator, S.N. and Bedrossian, J.L. (1988), *Communication Assessment and Intervention for Adults with Mental Retardation*, Taylor and Francis, London.

Carr, E.H. and Durand, M.V. (1985), 'The social-communicative basis of severe behaviour problems' in S. Reiss and R. Bootzin (eds), *Theoretical Issues in Behavior Therapy*, New York: Academic Press.

Carr, E.G. Levin, L., McConachie, G., Carlson, J.I., Kemp, D.C. and Smith, C.E. (1993), *Communication-based Intervention for Problem Behavior: A User's Guide for Producing Positive Change*, New York: Brooks Cole.

Department of Health (1993), *Services for People with Learning Disabilities and Challenging Behaviour or Mental Health Needs: Report of a Project Group* (Chair: Prof. J.L. Mansell), London: Department of Health.

Durand, M. V. (1990), *Functional Communication Training: An Intervention for Severe Behavior Problems*, New York: Guilford.

Joint Learning Disability Service (1997), *The Use of Massage and Aromatherapy for People with Learning Disabilities*, Manchester: Joint Learning Disability Service.

Jolliffe, J. (1996), *Comprehension Assessment Schedule*, Manchester: Mancunian Community Health NHS Trust.

Kiernan, C. and Qureshi, H. (1993), 'Challenging behaviour' in C. Kiernan (ed), *Research to Practice? Implications of Research on the Challenging Behaviour of People with Learning Disability*, Clevedon: BILD Publications.

Kiernan, C., Reid, B. and Goldbaft, J. (1987), *Foundations of Communication and Language*, Manchester: Manchester University Press/BIMH.

Lally, J., Menzies, S. and Low, K. (1995a), *How You Can Help: People with Both Learning Disabilities and Physical Disabilities*, Manchester: Joint Learning Disability Service.

Lally, J., Menzies, S. and Low, K. (1995b), *How You Can Help: People with Both Learning Disabilities and Visual Impairment and/or Hearing Impairment*, Manchester: Joint Learning Disability Service.

Maitland, S., Horne, R. and Burton M. (1996), 'An exploration of the Alexander Technique for people with learning disabilities', *British Journal of Learning Disabilities*, 24 (2), 70–76.

Paul, R. *et al.* (1987), 'A comparison of language characteristics of mentally retarded adults with fragile X syndrome and those with nonspecific retardation and autism', *Journal of Autism and Developmental Disorders*, 17, 457–68.

Peccei, J.S. (1994), *Child Language*, London: Routledge.

Reisman, J.E. and Hanschu, B. (1992), *Sensory Integration Inventory for Adults with Developmental Disabilities*, Minnesota: PDP Press.

Soper, G. and Robinson-Thorley, C. (1995), *MOTTO Sensory Approach*, Brentwood: BHB Community Care NHS Trust.

Speake, B. and Kellaway, M. (1992), 'Survey of adults using learning disability services in South Manchester', unpublished.

Tager-Flusberg, H. (1989), 'A psycholinguistic perspective on language development in the autistic child' in G. Dawson (ed.), *Autism: New Directions in Diagnosis, Nature, and Treatment in the Autistic Child*, New York: Guilford.

Tager-Flusberg, H., Calkins, S., Nolin, T., Bamberger, T., Anderson, M. and Chadwick-Dias, A. (1990), 'A longitudinal study of language acquisition in autistic and Down syndrome children', *Journal of Autism and Development Disorders*, 20, 1–21.

Van der Gaag, A. (1988), *Communication Assessment Profile for Adults with a Mental Handicap*, Bicester: Winslow.

Van der Gaag, A. and Dormandy, K. (1993), *Communication and Adults with Learning Disabilities*, London: Whurr.

10 Service response to sexual abuse of people with learning disabilities

Jude Moss and Christine Adcock

Introduction

The move to recognise and respect the sexual rights of people with learning disabilities has brought the issue of sexual abuse to the fore. Agencies that serve people with learning disabilities have begun to acknowledge their responsibilities to protect their users and to provide appropriate services to support survivors of abuse.

In Manchester policies and procedures have been developed that outline the service response to all aspects of abuse. It has been recognised that attention must be paid to enabling staff to help service users disclose incidents of abuse and recover from the distress it may have caused. This chapter discusses the Joint Service's attempt to begin to address the complex issue of people's emotional needs in this context.

Key issues

Definitions

Definition of sexual abuse is a complex issue. It raises issues of assessing consent, of making decisions about appropriate and inappropriate behaviour and forces consideration of complex issues such as non-contact abuse. These concerns must be addressed in the context of inequalities of power so pervasive that fundamental issues such as a person's sexual orientation and preferences are often ignored. Services in Manchester use the following definition:

Any form of sexual activity to which a person has not consented, or by virtue of their level of development, to which they are unable to give informed consent so that their apparent willingness has been exploited.

How much abuse is there?

Assessing the prevalence of sexual abuse of people with learning disabilities is particularly problematic, and estimates of prevalence vary widely, from 4–5 per cent (Cooke, 1989) to 37 per cent (Elvick *et al.*, 1990).

Data from a survey of reported sexual abuse by Turk and Brown (1992) suggests that, in a city like Manchester (with a population of just over 400 000) there would be between six and eight *reported* new victims per year. However, estimates depend on levels of awareness of abuse and on the definitions and methodology used.

In Turk and Brown's (1992) survey:

- although women were more likely to be abused, the proportion of male victims was greater than in the non-learning-disabled population
- victims had all levels of learning disability from profound to mild
- the vast majority of perpetrators of abuse were male and known and familiar to the individual
- a significant proportion of perpetrators were learning-disabled people
- in many cases, one perpetrator committed multiple offences
- most abuse took place in the homes of the victim or perpetrator, although other venues included day or leisure facilities and public places, such as parks and on public transport.

Despite some variations in the research literature, it is clear that sexual abuse is a reality for a great many learning-disabled people. There are also indications that they are more likely to suffer sexual abuse than the rest of the population.

Vulnerability factors

There are now strong pointers in the direction of mental handicap itself being a risk factor for all forms of child abuse including sexual abuse. (Vizard, 1989)

Why might learning-disabled people be more vulnerable to sexual abuse than the rest of the population? A number of factors can be suggested, relating to both the individual victims and to their environments. People with learning disabilities may have:

- little knowledge about sexuality
- poor communication skills to disclose or describe what has happened
- a higher level of dependence on others for intimate care
- higher levels of trust and suggestibility
- higher levels of compliance
- poor assertiveness and self defence skills
- poor understanding of the appropriateness of the behaviour of others.

Factors that relate to the environments in which people live may include:

- institutionalised settings
- being cared for by a succession of paid staff
- increased exposure to perpetrators – both to the learning-disabled people who abuse and to perpetrators who actively seek employment or contact with potential victims.

The attitudes held about learning-disabled people may create an environment in which abuse is more likely to take place:

- The common belief that learning-disabled people are not fully human implies that abusing them matters less.
- A belief exists that learning-disabled people's poor intellectual skills will somehow prevent them understanding or being hurt by their experience and that they won't understand, won't be damaged and won't complain.
- The stereotype of learning-disabled people being hypersexual may also reduce a perpetrator's inhibitions.

A service must be aware of all these issues when considering how to address the needs of its service users.

Effects

Although the literature on the impact of sexual abuse on learning-disabled people is relatively small, it suggests that the effects are consistent with those experienced by other survivors. Although each individual survivor of abuse is different, there seem to be some common experiences.

Typical survivors of abuse often report emotional experiences of betrayal, powerlessness, shame, anger and guilt. These feelings are often manifested through a range of behaviours, including withdrawal, aggression, self-harm, eating and sleeping disorders and many more. For learning-disabled people there may be additional or slightly different manifestations. Some of the effects may also be compounded by other aspects of the disability such as poor comprehension or communication skills, chronic low self-esteem and the lack of close supportive relationships.

Unfortunately, the way in which learning-disabled people express the impact and effects of sexual abuse are often labelled as challenging behaviour by a service that is unaware of how such people react to trauma. Eating and sleeping disorders may be attributed to physical illness, mood changes, aggression and isolation may be ignored, and self-injury and inappropriate sexual behaviour may be seen as being part of the disability itself. When these 'problems' are taken at face value and treated without an understanding of the underlying cause, they are likely to reoccur or the distress might be manifested in some other guise. As Fenwick (1994) asks, 'One cannot help but wonder just how many people with "challenging behaviour" have been victims of sexual abuse at some time in their lives?'

Behavioural change occurs for many reasons. Sexual abuse must be considered as one possible cause, but others must always be explored. Services need to guard against two types of error:

1   assuming sexual abuse has happened when it has not
2   assuming sexual abuse has not happened, when it has.

Practical guidance

Services have a responsibility to protect their users from abuse and to provide appropriate environments and therapeutic services for people who have experienced it.

Prevention

Prevention of abuse is a complex issue. There must be a multi-element approach to prevention that considers the individuals themselves within the culture of the service in which they live. The organisational culture must assume:

1   that every person is at risk, and
2   that the risk is so great that social and health care support must prioritise prevention and not see it as less important than responding to 'the crisis' when it has occurred.

The service

Some people with learning disabilities find it difficult to take full control over their lives, and much of their care and the decisions about their lives are made by service providers. Given this level of responsibility, it is imperative that the service takes positive action towards the prevention of abuse. This involves raising awareness within the service and giving clear messages to its staff and the people it serves that it is aware of sexual abuse and is not prepared to tolerate it. This can be progressed through devising effective policies, procedures, and associated training (see Chapter 6).

Such policies must explicitly have care of the individual at the core, rather than appearing primarily protective of the service. Staff should be in no doubt about what is acceptable and, if they have concerns, should be enabled and supported to 'whistle-blow' with no fear of retribution from the service. The discouragement of whistle-blowing is one of the most harmful attitudes of services in that it compounds the distress of both service users and front-line staff.

Once it is acknowledged that perpetrators of sexual abuse may actively seek out 'good' victims, it becomes clear how careful the service must be when employing staff. At interview, explicit statements and emphasis on abuse prevention procedures and guidelines give clear messages to potential perpetrators that the service does not provide a closed environment where abuse will go unnoticed or unchallenged. Services could also make a commitment to refrain from merely asking known perpetrators to resign from their service so that they can simply go and continue to abuse elsewhere.

The service must also acknowledge those activities that place individual service users in particularly vulnerable situations. Most obvious is the issue of intimate personal care. However, the process of writing policies about such care and ensuring they are followed at all times raises dilemmas and difficulties. For example, it is widely felt to be desirable for same-sex intimate care to occur when possible and with the highest degree of privacy possible but, in terms of abuse, we know that the vast majority of abusers are male and that male service users are also at risk. If protection was the sole aim of the service, employing female-only staff might be a good step, yet this conflicts with other elements of desirable service provision. Such issues must be carefully considered and, where risk occurs, there must be clear guidance and a system for ensuring that policies are followed and any problems quickly dealt with. The Joint Service tries to ameliorate some of the difficulties of same-sex cover, by using induction and other training to emphasise these values and has expectations that gender and intimacy issues are understood and responded to wherever possible.

Clearly, some sexual abuse is perpetrated by learning-disabled people. The service often takes the responsibility of choosing who people live with, with whom they spend their days and must therefore be prepared to protect service users from those learning-disabled people who are known, or suspected, to have assaulted others. There must be good risk assessment, options for moving people, flexible and effective supervision, and treatment for perpetrators to reduce future danger to others. Staff must be clear about what is acceptable and feel comfortable about tackling incidents that are either inappropriate or causing distress. All those working in the service need to be clear about the law and to be able to access legal guidance.

If the whole service acknowledges and addresses these complex issues, it can set the context for work with individuals that supports and values prevention, in order to reduce the need for crisis management when the damage is already done.

Individual service users

In terms of enabling individuals to prevent abuse taking place, good sex education is vital. It can facilitate knowledge of the physical body, provide a vocabulary with which to talk about sexual matters and give clear messages about people's right to their sexuality. It also demonstrates that the service recognises the importance of the sexuality of the people it serves. It is during sex education sessions that people feel enabled to disclose abuse that has occurred.

Social skills training is important, yet often neglected: it helps people understand and negotiate in the social world and includes important skills such as appropriate assertion and the making and ending of relationships (Burton and Kagan, 1995). Groups that enable people to explore assertiveness, parenthood and relationships are useful. Attention must be paid to increasing people's awareness of their rights and how to respond when those rights are not respected. Self-advocacy is a vital element of this.

Staff training

Staff training is a key element in prevention. Staff need to be trained to know exactly what is meant by sexual abuse, the risks, the likely perpetrators, the possible effects of abuse, the ways in which the service is tackling the issue and their role in the process. They also need to know what to do when supporting people whom they know or suspect have been abused. Effective policies and practice guidelines are invaluable in providing the platform from which sensitive prevention and intervention can occur. Only when staff feel safe can they allow themselves to 'hear' that service users are not safe and thus give permission for the service users to tell staff. From here the process of healing can begin.

The service has a responsibility to do all it can to prevent abuse and also to train itself to recognise and tackle abuse when it does take place. Equally important, however, are the approaches taken once abuse is known to have occurred.

Disclosure

In this context, we are referring to disclosure as the first time an individual 'tells' anyone that they have experienced abuse. This can be done in a number of different ways and is sometimes more appropriately seen as the time when we finally understand what a service user may have been telling us for a long time (see 'Effects', p. 163). At the disclosure stage there are a number of important issues to consider, alongside the proper procedures.

Abuse is least likely to be disclosed to those people within the service who have the most knowledge about the subject. Service users are most likely to disclose abuse to the front-line staff with whom they have built up close and trusting relationships. These staff therefore need to be aware of how disclosure may occur and of how best to respond when it does occur. The way in which the individual is treated at this point is crucial.

It is important for staff to have already considered the emotional reactions which they themselves might experience. The disbelief, disgust, anger and powerlessness which they might feel increase the probability that the disclosure will be ignored, belittled, disbelieved or challenged. Staff should therefore be given the opportunity, in the form of sensitive training, to work through these issues to some extent so that they will be able to handle disclosure in a way that does not compound the hurt already experienced by the individual. This may be particularly important if the alleged perpetrator is a colleague.

Towards an effective response: developments in Manchester

Intervention

One way of tackling the issue of intervention is to begin with the premise that different people need different levels of help and that to provide that help requires different levels of expertise. At the 'base of the triangle' are the needs that all victims have that can be addressed by all those around them. In Manchester, we are developing and implementing a strategic plan to try to build a training and supervision strategy which involves the following:

- Module 1: General training for front-line staff in basic counselling skills.
- Module 2: Training on how to use these skills when a person is disclosing, or has disclosed, abuse.
- Module 3: Development of a group of 'dedicated' workers who receive support and supervision to help staff and service users through a specific incident and its effects.

This will support the current training available to all staff on the service policies and procedures, which includes a great deal of introductory information on the subject of abuse.

Level one needs

The first strand of the strategy is to give front-line staff a repertoire of counselling skills for use with anyone in distress. Basic counselling skills are a prerequisite for all the work required in this area. Direct care staff often seem frightened to address the issue of abuse with people whom they support on account of not knowing what to do. Sexual abuse is such a complex and emotive issue that it seems to require an expert to deal with it. The fear may be that doing anything will make it worse. However, we feel that, like any form of physical harm, the damage and hurt caused by sexual abuse can heal naturally if the person is in an environment which promotes and facilitates that healing process. This can be a very helpful notion for staff if they are helped first to understand the damage caused by abuse and then realise that they have a role in creating a 'healing' environment by acting as a supporter and advocate rather than as some kind of therapist. Staff need basic counselling skills so that they can listen to the account of the abuse without giving advice, reassuring or trying to undermine the other person's feelings. This is extremely difficult to do without some level of training. Staff must understand that making it clear to the individual that they are believed can be an extremely powerful healing experience in itself.

In the basic counselling skills training we have used a format of *active listening*, using the concepts of empathy, warmth and genuineness but have tried to help people understand the psychodynamic notion of *countertransference* as well. We extended the training in this way to help staff respond to people whose verbal abilities are extremely limited. In this, we have made the assumption (following Sinason, 1992) that learning-disabled people can have a high 'emotional intelligence' even when their intellectual abilities are restricted and that people with little or no verbal ability should have access to counselling processes. So we took a pragmatic decision to mix active listening skills, plus some ways of reading body language, plus a very simple understanding of countertransference. We try to explain that in sitting or being with a person with learning disabilities, part of what you feel is the feelings generated by yourself (anxiety at getting it wrong, pressures of the work rota and so on) part of it is between you and the service user (empathy, sadness, upset) and part of it is a direct *emotional* communication from the learning-disabled person. In other words we encourage staff, to entertain the possibility that if they are feeling anxious, scared and angry, this may not just be to do with them, but may be a *direct* and precise communication from the service user of his or her feelings. This happens with no words exchanged and can be commented on. Staff find this concept difficult to accept but, once grasped, it is very powerful. If they are mistaken, the other person will let them know and, as long as the interpretation has been offered gently, will not put up barriers. If they are right, it can give so much to the learning-disabled person – that wonderful relief of not being alone, being understood, of having someone make that effort. This experience of someone letting us know what something has truly been like for us is rare, but it is even rarer for someone with a learning disability. The skill for staff is to understand what is in them, what is in the person being counselled and what is a communication from one to the other.

Morris (1992) describes the tasks of the advocate/carer throughout the process of healing. Initially it is to be a witness, to acknowledge the reality of the abuse, then to spend time with the survivor, supporting them while they make some sort of sense of the abuse. They must also support the survivor's progression of feelings that might change from despair to mourning to rage. Accepting these feelings is vital, as even subtle messages that grief and anger are unbearable or unacceptable will further halt the healing process. The advocate may be able to encourage the release of emotion or devise creative ways of releasing anger. Obviously there co-exists with these tasks the need for staff to have access to good support networks. In some sense, their task is to bear the experience for the individual, and to believe and accept what the person is saying as the reality. The emotion aroused by this is important because, if support is not given and the staff's emotional reactions dealt with appropriately, the experience of the abuse victim is likely to be very negative and further damage could be done. Some people may falsely report abuse, and it is important that staff 'listen' to the emotional communication rather than merely judge whether or not the incident occurred. In Manchester, the Joint Service has planned to provide further training to front-line staff who have already achieved a certain level of basic competence so that they can explore in more detail those complex issues of using counselling skills when someone has been abused.

All this training should be within a context that is supportive of staff who have to respond to these emotionally taxing matters. Staff who are not having their own needs for support met, and are angry and confused, are unlikely to be able to deal with the anger and confusion of the people they support.

The role of the staff is also to ensure that, within the environment in which the person lives and works, there are good working practices and consistency of messages. For example, there is little point in an abused client receiving help around issues of privacy and assertiveness for an hour a week if, when they get home, those needs are not also respected. Staff need to be helped to feel competent and to realise that, with a minimum of training, there is very little they could do to make the situation worse and a great deal they could do to support the person well.

If the staff have been enabled to have an understanding of the possible effects of sexual abuse they will be unlikely to seek inappropriate 'help' for the symptoms they see. For example, if they are aware that eating and sleeping disturbances can be symptoms of abuse, they are less likely to assume that it is merely a medical problem. Similarly, if the expression of confusion or rage is understood as a natural part of recovery from trauma then they will probably respond more sensitively to behavioural outbursts, rather than simply develop a behavioural programme to eradicate them or dismiss them as 'attention-seeking'.

This is the basic level of support that all people need to carry out the long process of recovery. The timescale of this process should not be underestimated. Once all the procedures have been followed, the survivor stands at the beginning of their own process of recovery – a process in which the direct care staff can play a fundamental role.

Level two needs

The effects of sexual abuse will be different for each individual, and their recovery will be very much determined not only by the environment in which they live and work but also by their prior experiences, their coping strategies and psychological defences. For this reason, some people need specialised expert care to enable them to integrate their experiences, accept them, recover and move on. There has been relatively little written about this, and many clinicians are 'feeling their way' while working with clients, adapting what few techniques and methods are described in the small body of literature. These reports are varied and reflect the diversity of psychotherapeutic approaches. For these reasons, we are making links with specialised therapeutic services that can offer long-term therapy. We are doing this in three ways:

1 by developing contacts and working relationships with services for people who are not learning-disabled and who have been abused (both specialised psychotherapeutic services and with the independent sector – for example, survivors groups and rape crisis centres)
2 by training existing practitioners in individual therapeutic work, and by receiving supervision from psychotherapists who specifically work with learning-disabled people
3 by developing, within Manchester, a group of people with counselling experience who will receive external, specialist supervision and training so that they can support service users and staff intensively through specific incidents.

The literature on therapy for survivors offers some useful ideas on the different approaches that might also prove valuable. One such approach is group therapy. Often the basic remit of group therapy for survivors of sexual abuse is to try and redress the imbalance of power that pervades the individual's lives and led to the abuse. To this end, groups are often facilitated rather than led, have clarity around the issues of boundaries and respect, and involve group members having to share the responsibility and power of the group. The therapeutic aspects within the group often centre round the issues mentioned in the section on level one needs, bearing witness to an individual's pain, supporting and allowing expression of emotion. A group can be a good arena for the learning of new coping skills, relaxation and other therapeutic techniques and exercises.

Other useful approaches are based on cognitive behavioural interventions, focusing on the specific emotional and cognitive processing problems resulting from trauma. There is also valuable case material written from a psychoanalytic perspective. As with the wider population, some individuals are most effectively helped through such individual psychotherapy. For many years this has not been an option available to learning-disabled people, partly because it was thought that verbal skills were required to make use of it. However, in recent years there have been small pockets of work, primarily that done by Sinason, showing clearly that psychotherapy can be a powerful therapeutic tool for survivors of abuse who have learning disabilities. At present, resources are incredibly scarce, with few training opportunities. However, if it is through these specialised services that people who have received numerous unsuccessful behavioural or other approaches are actually able to begin to recover from trauma then it is important that we take the lack of access seriously and try to begin to rectify the situation.

A service must also address the complex issue of working with those who are survivors of abuse, but who themselves abuse. Their needs must be recognised and fulfilled both as individuals in their own right but also to protect other people. Again, the work that has been done in this area is at an early developmental level but should be acknowledged as a priority by any service.

Conclusion

This chapter has attempted a definition of sexual abuse and explored the complexity of consent and the quality of the power relationship. It demonstrated how vulnerable people with a learning disability can be, because of their functional abilities, the environment in which they live, their dependence on others for support, and the myths and misconceptions about their sexuality and feelings. It also likens the impact of sexual abuse on learning-disabled people to that experienced by anyone, but often compounded by poor comprehension, poor communication and chronic low self-esteem.

Services are encouraged to concentrate on preventing abuse. Awareness training for staff, explicit policies, careful recruitment and protection 'whistle-blowers' will create a culture where abuse is both recognised and not tolerated. Sex education and social skills training will help empower the service users.

This chapter has described an approach to training which will provide the opportunity for the healing to begin from the point of disclosure. It advocates a structured initiative which equips direct care staff with basic counselling skills. The positive message is that, with a minimum of training, there is very little that staff can do to make a situation worse and a great deal that they could do to support the person well.

The chapter concludes by sharing the experience of clinicians who have tried to develop more specialised skills.

References and resources

Burton, M. and Kagan, C.M. (1995), *Social Skills for People with Learning Disabilities: A Social Capability Approach*, London: Chapman and Hall.

Cooke, L.B. (1989), 'Abuse of mentally handicapped adults', *British Medical Journal*, 299–392.

Elvick, S.L., Berkowitz, C.D., Nicholas, E., Lipman, J.L. and Inkelis, S.H. (1990), 'Sexual abuse in the developmentally disabled: dilemmas in diagnosis', *Child Abuse and Neglect*, **14**, 497–502.

Fenwick, A. (1994), 'Sexual abuse in adults with learning disabilities. Part 1: A review of the literature', *British Journal of Learning Disabilities*, 22, 53–6.

Finkelhor, D. and Hotaling, G.T. (1984), 'Sexual abuse in the National Incidence Study of child abuse and neglect: an appraisal', *Child Abuse and Neglect*, 8, 23–33.

Morris, S. (1992), 'Responding to sexual abuse', *NAPSAC Bulletin* (2), 6–9.

Sinason V. (1992), *Mental Handicap and the Human Condition. New Approaches from the Tavistock*, London: Free Association Books.

Turk ,V. and Brown, H. (1992), 'Sexual abuse and adults with learning disabilities', *Mental Handicap*, 20, 56–8.

Vizard, E. (1989), 'Child sexual abuse and mental handicap: a child psychiatrist's perspective', in H. Brown and A. Craft (eds), *Thinking the Unthinkable*, London: FPA Education Unit.

11 Prevention of challenging behaviour and service user distress

Jean Lally

Introduction

Imagine you are a manager sitting at your desk late on a Friday afternoon. You have had an extremely busy week. The phone rings. A member of your staff tells you that a service user in a residential house has attacked them seriously. You have to go out to sort out the situation. The service user has become upset, the member of staff is distressed, and you need to support both of them when you have many competing demands on your time.

What exactly might have been done to prevent distress to everyone concerned? This chapter outlines some ideas to empower hands-on staff to act to lessen the likelihood of situations like this.

Key issues

How can staff help prevent challenging behaviour?

Staff need to attend to the signs that the service user is not content

Someone may show signs that they are not content – they may be in pain, ill, unhappy, uncomfortable, anxious, angry and so on. Aggression can therefore sometimes be prevented by changing the situation so that the person no longer experiences these sensations or emotions. Staff need to know how a service user demonstrates their unhappiness. They need to act as quickly as possible and/or plan to prevent discontent before it builds up to a level where aggression may be aroused. This requires particular sensitivity in cases where the person finds it difficult to communicate how they feel. Of course, even if the person does not show aggressive behaviour, and does not complain strongly, good quality of care means attending to the signs and causes of discontent and making the person's life happier.

Staff need to learn to identify and attend to the cause of distress

As we know from our own lives, distress can be due to an enormous number of causes which can vary from day to day. Aggression can occur because of numerous factors (which may individually be trivial) which have built up on a particular occasion to create a strong feeling of discontent. Staff therefore need to be constantly sensitive to a wide range of possible causes of distress in the people they support. Because staff in specialist teams are a scarce resource and cannot be constantly present to carry out this work, it is therefore vital to empower hands-on staff to be as effective as possible themselves.

However, staff may not be aware of important causes of aggressive behaviour and, if this is the case, they will not attend to them, report them to others or record them (for instance, in ABC charts). This means that no one will be able to prevent or attend to the service user's distressed state.

It has been suggested that staff may not attend effectively to the causes of challenging behaviour because of their emotional reactions to that behaviour (Bromley and Emerson, 1995). Therefore, where possible, it is preferable to encourage staff to attend to the cause *before* the person shows behavioural challenges – when the service user shows verbal or non-verbal signs of distress or/and by planning ahead to prevent likely distress.

Staff need to work with the person they support to help make their whole life as enjoyable and meaningful as possible

As Lovett (1996) emphasises, management has to support staff in this fundamental process of caring. He also explores the provocative questions: 'Who really cares for the person in the way that partners, relatives and friends can care for us?'; 'What may the person have to lose by showing challenging behaviour if nobody cares for their happiness outside of paid time?' From his perspective, preventing challenging behaviour means helping the person to develop a life in which they have activities and relationships which are as deep and sustaining as other people's.

Practical guidance

How can staff learn to attend to the signs that a person may not feel contented?

Staff need to know how people signal distress in general. They also need to know in detail the way in which a particular individual tends to signal distress – physical pain or internal emotional pain (for example, anxiety). A person who cannot speak often signals internal physical pain by banging the part that hurts – for example, they may hit their stomach when constipated. Internal emotional pain, such as anxiety, may be shown by the person's hands suddenly stiffening, for example. This action may be seen or felt by staff.

How can staff best attend to possible causes of distress?

Staff need to consider the environmental factors which may affect a particular person's level of internal distress in a range of situations. This can be deduced from:

1 *A knowledge of the person* (for example, they dislike meeting strangers). Essential lifestyle planning can be an invaluable help in giving a detailed knowledge of the person (see Chapter 17).
2 *A knowledge of situations.* People generally tend to dislike failure, they may be averse to carrying out activities which they find difficult.

It is necessary to know how to relate signs of distress to situations. For instance, one person who could not speak repeatedly banged his mouth and then walked to the telephone, and pointed at it. It emerged that his teeth hurt and he wanted staff to phone the dentist.

It is often useful to take into consideration past, as well as present, events. Staff need to communicate with the person (where possible) and others to find out what has happened in the person's recent or far past which might affect current situations. An empathic understanding can help make sense of previously perplexing behaviour.

Some broad categories of causes: demand, attention or physical problems

Causes of behavioural challenges can be very varied. Considerable research has been carried out to investigate challenging behaviour in the following circumstances: demand (where a person is asked to do something, sometimes in a teaching situation); lack of attention, being given attention when it is not wanted or for physical reasons (Carr, 1977; Carr and Durand, 1985). This research has tended to focus on people who speak very little, particularly those who self-injure.

To consider a demand situation, for example: a person might find a demand situation aversive for a wide variety of reasons. In each case they may show challenging behaviour in order to avoid or escape the situation. For example:

- A person with cerebral palsy becomes anxious when asked to take part in a tabletop activity because, when they bend forward to take part in the activity, they are afraid that they might fall out of their wheelchair.
- A person may not understand what they have been asked to do – they do not understand words which describe actions and are only able to respond to gestures showing them what to do. They therefore become confused and anxious.
- A person's hearing aid is clogged with wax and so they do not hear the request. Again, they may begin to find the situation threatening.
- A person is in physical pain (say, from impacted constipation) and therefore feels generally irritable and aggressive. He then repeatedly bites an acupressure point (Lovett, 1996).

Attending to the cause

The demand situations described above can be looked at in relation to prevention. For instance, if staff know how and when to use gestures to help the person understand what they want, the person may not then find the demand situation aversive. If staff know that a woman feels pain during menstruation and is happier, at that time, lying down, having taken paracetamol rather than being asked to go horse-riding, they will not ask her to participate on that occasion (although she would be asked and encouraged to take part at other times, because it is known that she generally enjoys the activity and therefore does not want to avoid it).

Knowing how to help can prevent or reduce challenging behaviour. If carers attend to causes *before* a person shows challenging behaviour – by reacting to early signs of distress and/or by planning ahead to make a situation less aversive – there will be no reason for challenging behaviour to develop. If the function of the challenging behaviour is to avoid a situation, and the person no longer wishes to avoid it, they do not need to show challenging behaviour. It has been prevented.

Emerson (1995) concludes that the type of approach which focuses on changing the antecedents or context of challenging behaviour is relatively easy to implement and sustain over time, with no negative side-effects being reported in the literature. We suggest, in this chapter, that effective prevention consists of applying the same type of antecedent/context approach in very specific ways *before* challenging behaviour develops. The situation should be considered in relation to the person's wider pattern of life – for example, their reaction to a particular situation may be a result of a general experience of little being interesting or enjoyable. Furthermore, specific situations should be considered in terms of the sense they make for the person's wider pattern of experience. For example, are the demands being made for the person's benefit or not? There is a subtle ethical debate here, as we all have to adapt to the demands of others. However, if someone is obviously not enjoying an activity it is always useful to ask the following 'so what?' question:

Will the person's life be improved by taking part in this activity, either now or in the future?

This approach is even more important when the person can't tell us what is upsetting them.

Challenging behaviour is thought often to have a communicative function. The more we can attend to a person's distressed states in the way described above, the less will the person need to communicate through challenging behaviour. This approach will help the person even in cases where they do not signal distress through challenging behaviour. For instance, physical signs of sexual abuse (past or present) need to be identified and appropriate therapy sought.

Moreover, even people who can communicate verbally do not always do so. Such service users should be enabled and encouraged to communicate verbally any distress and the reasons for it.

Planning ahead to reduce likely causes of aversiveness

Burton and Jones (see Chapter 12) and Felce (1989) describe how environments can be structured to lessen the likelihood of service user challenging behaviour. Essential Lifestyle Planning (see Chapter 17) can also be used to prompt staff to plan to reduce the likelihood of the person becoming distressed.

Examples from Manchester

The research project

How much do front-line staff know about the causes of service users' distress? In a pilot study, 24 newly employed residential social workers in the Joint Service were assessed on their awareness of a range of specific antecedents to service user distress. Staff said that they did not know, or had not considered, the information covered in a mean of 11 out of 81 questions (range 0–35). These figures are likely to be an underestimate because staff may not have wished to admit that they did not know information. (Interestingly, several staff also volunteered that the questionnaire had helped remind them of information they had forgotten.)

Consultation with professionals

After consultation, professionals in a community team identified a number of factors which they thought, from their experience, were important in affecting service users' distress and which they thought hands-on staff did not necessarily know about and therefore could not observe.

Series of booklets

As a result of the research project and consultation, it was decided to produce a series of booklets (20–30 A5 pages each) which would not only bring to staff attention factors of which they might be unaware but would also help them prevent challenging behaviour with learning-disabled people in the manner suggested above. The booklets were also to inform staff how to identify when a person was distressed or found a situation aversive. It was intended that the booklets should cover the following topics:

1　physical disability (mainly cerebral palsy)
2　visual and hearing impairment
3　communication difficulties – difficulties in getting a message across
4　communication difficulties – difficulties in understanding
5　teaching (including demand and low-activity situations)
6　physical illness (for example, diabetes, thyroid problems)
7　feelings (in relation to change, abuse, bereavement and so on and to be produced after consultation with service users)
8　side-effects of medication
9　social relationships

10   how and what to observe and how to test ideas
11   psychological factors (including functional analysis).

The first four booklets have been produced in collaboration with a physio-therapist, nurse and speech and language therapist. They are used in the Joint Service. Others are being prepared. People First in Manchester have contributed ideas in the preparation of two of the booklets and are to be consulted regarding the others.

The booklets are designed to help service staff in a variety of challenging behaviour as detailed below.

Preventing challenging behaviour which is due to the service user wishing to avoid demands

Many factors which may affect demand situations are mentioned in the booklets, including those mentioned on p. 178.

Preventing challenging behaviour which is due to the service user wishing to avoid attention

Figure 11.1 illustrates some techniques which might help in a case where someone wishes to avoid attention. Appropriate techniques like these could prevent the onset of challenging behaviour being shown, by reducing the aversiveness of the situation.

If the staff member is approaching the person in a way that they can tolerate the person will not want to avoid this attention. Challenging be-haviour will not have a function and will not appear. Challenging behav-iour will therefore have been prevented.

Preventing challenging behaviour which is due to the person seeking attention

A service user may seek attention for a wide variety of reasons. For in-stance, someone may have a pain that needs attending to. When a person seeks attention in these circumstances staff should respond immediately, identify the pain and take action wherever possible *before* challenging be-haviour is shown. If the person's needs are met early enough, challenging behaviour will no longer have a function. The ways in which service users may signal pain have been included in the booklets so that staff know what to look for.

☹ WHAT HURTS: BEING SPOKEN TO WHEN YOU FIND SPEECH UPSETTING.	☺ HOW YOU CAN HELP THESE PEOPLE TO FIND IT LESS STRESSFUL WHEN OTHERS TALK TO THEM
Have you ever been in the situation when you were sitting quietly in a pleasant daydream and somebody rudely shattered your peace, leaving you feeling nervous and resentful?	* **Give a warning** that you are going to interact with the person – Sit beside them or stand near them, wait until they look at you and then say their name quietly.
A few people, particularly those people labelled autistic, find it distressing to be spoken to. They may shout "Leave me alone! Leave me alone! **Leave me alone**!" They find the world a confusing place, and they easily become anxious. They feel calmest when they are alone in situations they know well.	* **Use short sentences. If you don't need to say anything – don't!** You may often be able to interact in silence. * **Wait after you have spoken** for the person to adjust to the disturbance and calm down. They may then respond to you.
Unfortunately, by refusing to spend time with other people, these individuals may miss out on experiences that they would very much enjoy.	* After a pause, **repeat** what you said calmly. * **Use pictures instead of words** wherever possible. For instance, you could show the person a photo of the park, rather than saying "Would you like to go to the park?"

Source: Jolliffe and Lally, 1997.

Figure 11.1 Extract from booklet

Subject-matter and layout of the booklets

'References and Resources' (see pp. 184–5) gives a list of titles and shows the range of situations which are covered. More booklets can be produced as required.

The layout of each booklet is such that preventive strategies and/or who to contact for more details (on the right-hand page) are shown clearly in relation to each cause (on the left-hand page). Figure 11.1 (p. 182) illustrates this, although the typing is smaller in the figure and the whole page is not shown.

Throughout the booklets:

- staff are encouraged to empathise with the service user's situation (see Figure 11.1. 'Have you ever been in a situation when you were sitting quietly ...?').
- staff are referred to specialists for more help in situations where they are unable to apply preventive techniques adequately on their own.

It is intended to continually update the booklets so that they form a flexible and comprehensive reference package for hands-on staff and managers.

Initial feedback has been very positive. For instance, in one house where a service user was losing her sight, staff redesigned the environment and were stimulated to contact a local organisation for more help. Staff found the booklets clear and easy to read, and volunteered that they increased empathy. People First and individual service users have approved strongly. A family placement carer added detail to the booklets, specific to the person she supported. She then gave them to support workers to read, so that they might better understand and help that person. She also noted that the format of the booklets was more accessible and acceptable than a professional report might be. Appraisal of new staff has shown that staff need to know, or be reminded of, the information contained in the booklets.

The booklets are to be given to all new staff as soon as they start work, in addition to being available in the residential networks and for community team members. Information in the booklets is backed up by a comprehensive staff training system.

Currently, ways in which staff can best learn and be motivated to apply the information in the booklets are being developed.

Conclusion

This chapter has described an approach to the prevention of both service user distress and challenging behaviour:

- Observe signs of service user distress.
- Identify the possible causes of the distress.
- Attend to those causes.

There is scope for considerable research, investigating how to make the approach most effective in practice. For instance, what helps or hinders staff in observing signs of service user distress? What motivates staff to attend to signs of distress *before* behavioural problems occur?

It is essential that staff are *continually sensitive* to signs that the service user may be becoming distressed and that they try to lessen the reasons for this distress. Forward planning can reduce the likelihood of service users being placed in situations which they find aversive.

The chapter has also given detail of booklets produced in Manchester which can be a useful tool in assisting hands-on staff to apply the approach more effectively, with help from specialist staff in some cases.

Not all challenging behaviour can be prevented because, in this imperfect world, it is an impossible task to control all its causes. However, if this approach is applied, the frequency and intensity of challenging behaviour are likely to be reduced, and crises such as the one mentioned at the beginning of this chapter should be less likely to occur.

References and resources

Bromley, J. and Emerson, E. (1995), 'Beliefs and emotional reactions of care staff working with people with challenging behaviour', *Journal of Intellectual Disability Research*, **39**, 341–52.
Carr, E.G. (1977), 'The motivation of self-injurious behaviour: a review of some hypotheses', *Psychological Bulletin*, **84**, 800–816.
Carr, E.G. and Durand, V.M. (1985), 'The social–communicative basis of severe behaviour problems in children' in: S. Reiss and R. Bootzin (eds), *Theoretical Issues in Behavior Therapy*, New York: Academic Press, 219–54.
Emerson, E (1995), *Challenging behaviour: Analysis and Intervention in People with Learning Difficulties*, Cambridge: Cambridge University Press.
Felce, D. (1989), *Staffed Housing for Adults with Severe or Profound Mental Handicaps: The Andover Project*, Kidderminster: BIMH Publications.
Lovett, H. (1996), *Learning to Listen*, Baltimore: Paul Brookes.

The *How You can Help* series of booklets

Jolliffe, J. and Lally, J. (1997), *How You can Help: People with Both Learning Disabilities and Communication Difficulties. Difficulties in Getting a Message Across*, Manchester: Joint Learning Disability Service.

Joliffe, J. and Lally, J. (1997), *How You can Help: People with Both Learning Disabilities and Communication Difficulties. Difficulties in Understanding*, Manchester: Joint Learning Disability Service.

Lally, J., Menzies, S. and Low, K. (1995), *How You can Help: People with Both Learning Disabilities and Physical Disabilities*, Manchester: Joint Learning Disability Service.

Lally, J., Menzies, S. and Low, K. (1995), *How You can Help. People with Both Learning Disabilities and Visual Impairment and/or Hearing Impairment*, Manchester: Joint Learning Disability Service.

12 Developing effective provision for people who may present behavioural challenges: clinically managed social care

Mark Burton and Phil Jones

Introduction

A significant proportion of learning-disabled people at some time display behaviour that presents a challenge to themselves, others and the services provided. Estimates vary widely (17–56 per cent, according to Beange and Bauman, 1990); in an 'average health district' (population 220 000) 42 people might be expected to present serious challenging behaviour according to research carried out in the North West by Kiernan and Qureshi (1993). The move towards supported ordinary living in the community has highlighted the need for effective services provided locally.

Fifteen years ago, before the advent of the hospital resettlement and closure programmes, it was possible to make the rather crude assumption that behaviour problems were the result of living in unsatisfactory institutional environments. It was assumed that, once people were living in smaller-scale environments with good staffing ratios, behavioural problems would reduce considerably. Today, our understanding is rather more sophisticated. Without denying the effects of institutional life, it is now recognised that this is not the only cause of challenging behaviour. There is now a greater understanding that behavioural challenges are best understood as an interaction between three sets of factors:

1 **Individual factors.** Examples include: difficulties in communicating; difficulties in understanding things that happen; discomfort.
2 **Factors in the person's development and history.** Examples include: previous abuse; previous failure; lack of opportunity to learn relevant skills or acquire relevant knowledge.

3   **Factors in the present situation**. Examples include: social or task de-
    mands that exceed the person's skill or confidence; thwarting of wants
    and needs; noise levels.

Unfortunately, some of these factors, and some of the combinations between them, can be rather unexpected. This is especially so for staff who
work mainly on the basis of 'common sense', rather than on a combination
of 'good sense, additional knowledge, and problem-solving strategies'.

Learning disability services have always been staffed by a mixture of
qualified and unqualified staff. The newer community-based services have
tended to have particularly high levels of unqualified staff, both in local
authorities and the independent sector. This contrasts with the hospitals
where unqualified staff worked under the leadership of qualified staff. For
many people with learning disabilities – perhaps the majority – a great deal
can be achieved through providing opportunities, purpose and empathic
and practical support. However, this reaches its limits with people who
have complex and often counterintuitive needs.

The growth of community provision has led to an increase in professional staff working in the community. However, these have typically been
based in community teams, separated from the 'hard services' which provide home and daytime support to people. The professional staff often have
considerable skills in analysis and intervention with behavioural problems.
They work in an advisory capacity, depending on the cooperation of staff
and management who may not fully understand the basis for their recommendations. Moreover, professionals can be isolated from the day-to-day,
minute-by-minute pressures of life in the 'hard' services, and therefore
make recommendations that are difficult to follow, or which miss vital
aspects.

The question then arises:

*How do we get the skills to the point of service delivery without compromising the
ordinariness of the model of living in the community?*

This chapter identifies some of the issues to consider in providing for the
people who can present the most serious behavioural challenges, and also
describes the model that has developed in Manchester.

Key issues and practical guidance

Ordinary and complex needs

It is essential to recognise the full range of needs that people have. In Chapter 1 we distinguished between ordinary and special, or additional, needs (strictly speaking, these should be regarded as 'need satisfiers', Doyal and Gough, 1984, 1991). For those who may present behavioural challenges, we can broadly describe some of them as follows:

Ordinary needs
- Nutritious food.
- A comfortable house.
- People that know, understand and care.
- Being in ordinary places in the community.
- A guaranteed income.
- A unique and authentic identity.
- Purposeful activities.
- A sense of security and safety.

Special needs
- Help to understand and overcome behavioural problems, including expert investigation and the design and delivery of humane and effective interventions.
- Protection from dangers that are not understood, or arise from instances of behaviour.
- Effective teaching of new skills.
- A clear approach, shared by all care givers, that is continuously reviewed.
- Negotiation, and mediation, so that ordinary activities can be accessed without becoming threatening, unsafe, or stigmatising.

Some strange things can happen when either set of needs is neglected, as when services focus their efforts on one kind of need rather than the other. This can be demonstrated with a matrix as shown in Figure 12.1. The top left quadrant is relatively easy to identify, although services have tended to engage in fruitless debate between the top right and bottom left approaches. However, bringing about such a 'not only but also' approach does present some real difficulties, and constant vigilance is required to ensure an appropriate balance between the ordinary and special aspects.

	Ordinary needs met	Ordinary needs not met
Additional needs met	There is an overall agenda of addressing ordinary needs. Specialist knowledge, analysis, and intervention (for example, therapy, training, environmental structuring) are judiciously applied to support and enhance the person's inclusion in the routines, purposes, interactions and relationships of everyday life. The result is that the person's identity is respected, supported, and developed. Ethical safeguards consist of embedded expectations and norms within the culture of the service *and* formal process and procedures for review and decision-making.	Services are depersonalised and 'clinical', typically isolated from the patterns and meanings of everyday life. Technologies of behaviour change are applied, but without clarity about purposes (beyond behaviour change itself). There is reliance on the use of organisational power to ensure compliance, and great difficulty in embedding the maintenance of progress within the routines, purposes, interactions and relationships of everyday life. Ethical safeguards are likely to be weak in such environments.
Additional needs not met	Well intentioned attempts at inclusion fail, discrediting such approaches and legitimating approaches in the top right quadrant. Typically, behaviour problems continue and the person is given little or no appropriate help in overcoming them, staff become disillusioned, and there is a danger of blaming the person. Because the simplistic 'ordinary needs' orientation is allied to a strong ethical stance, the development of meaningful ethical safeguards is delayed since the service believes its design and goodwill is sufficient.	Neglect, abandonment, institutionalisation, total denial of human value. Strong likelihood of abuse. There are no safeguards beyond the concern of ordinary and active citizens.

Figure 12.1   Needs matrix

Synergy of approaches

Approaches to people presenting behavioural challenges have often been faddish. People who hurt themselves, attack others, or engage in bizarre health and safety-threatening behaviours can challenge our understanding and our abilities to work in a considered and effective way. As a result, there can be a tendency to look for the 'quick fix', or at least to oversimplify the issues. As a result, one theoretical framework (for example, behaviour analysis, communication, motor disorders, organic determinants) is followed while neglecting others.

Any one orientation is most unlikely to provide either an adequate understanding of behavioural problems or a universal practical approach. This means being prepared to use a variety of approaches, in an intelligent way, so that they mutually support one another.

To illustrate:

- Behavioural or functional analysis provides a useful framework for isolating some of the causes of behavioural challenges. It also allows the design of interventions for particular behaviours.
- 'Gentle teaching' provides useful ideas about establishing effective working relationships with people who challenge, and alerts us to the dangers of the abuse of power and control.
- Medical approaches help us to exclude and treat physical causes of behaviour problems (such as pain, disease, drug side-effects).
- Developmental approaches help us understand that the person's behaviours, abilities, and experiences are linked in an ordered and structured way. For example, developmental theory can help to understand some of the difficulty a person may experience when asked to participate in tasks they find too demanding.
- Communicative approaches help us to better mediate environmental events with people whose understanding and language may be limited.
- Philosophies of non-violence, together with the practice of self-defence, can help staff protect service users and themselves from physical harm.
- Social and organisational approaches help us to help staff teams work together effectively in coherently supporting someone with significant needs and challenges.
- Psychotherapeutic approaches help us understand the consequences of past trauma, and the impact on staff of supporting people with extreme and multiple needs.

It is our assertion that the best practice is informed by the combination of approaches, but that this must be backed by some idea of the appropriate scope and limits of each.

Establishing priorities

In working with people whose needs have not been met effectively up until now, an order of work typically emerges.

Initially, it is often important to establish control of the situation. This means establishing clear guidance for staff and setting clear boundaries for the service user. Given the extremity of some behaviour patterns this can mean prioritising some things over others. Choice, for example, can be a negative influence if allowed full rein at this stage: it may be important to establish a balanced diet, restrict caffeine or prevent bingeing by restricting free access to food stores. At the same time, safe practices need to be established, particularly if aggression is frequent, or likely, as boundaries are established. Services need effective policies and procedures for assessing and managing risk, as well as responding to violence and aggression, including the use of physical intervention (Coates, 1994; Harris, *et al.*, 1996).

For people who have been very withdrawn, or who have responded aggressively to requests to do things, it is important to begin establishing tolerance of another person's presence. Subsequently, it is essential to begin building up purposeful activity. The key here is to find a way of working with the person whereby demands are reduced, but some actions are performed. It may be important to start in a small way – for example, with one minute of dusting or even an arbitrary activity such as putting sponges into a bucket. It is often helpful to minimise the use of spoken language, and rely on imitation or gesture, and, where the person will accept them, physical prompts and guidance.

As the person becomes used to the boundaries, and to the security of predictable activities and staff reactions, it will be possible to extend activities and build up choice, or at least the person's involvement in selecting activities. A context for social interactions and communication is created, and this can be developed, again in a piecemeal fashion. Our best experience is that, in this process, which can take months or years, various critical points are reached – for example, as the person begins to talk about past experiences, or makes requests for things previously rejected, or becomes more tolerant to changes or delays.

Avoiding isolation and utilising management capacity

Setting up provision for people who present significant challenges is likely to take place within the context of larger service organisations. Even where a new piece of the service is created (for example, a house for one person or a small group), it is rarely free-standing. It is worth building on this fact to prevent isolation and to use resources effectively.

There is a danger of making the expertise that develops in work with the people with the biggest challenges inaccessible to the rest of the service. The opposite error lies in overloading this resource so that it cannot focus sufficiently on its primary task. To avoid falling into either trap, the boundary must be managed effectively. There is also a further danger of the specialist provision becoming out of touch with developments in the rest of the service even though these developments may be very relevant to meeting 'ordinary needs' effectively.

Finally, if a small and specialised service tries to be too self-sufficient it is likely to struggle with things such as sickness cover, and its skilled staff are likely to find themselves spending a great deal of time on matters such as housing management and repairs. It will often be better to draw on the wider service for the assistance that it can provide, while being self-sufficient in the things that it does not have available.

Given the dangers of such provision drifting to focus on special needs to the exclusion of ordinary ones, it is worth ensuring that the specialised service works to the same quality standards and policies as the rest of the service. Likewise, staff should have access to the same training opportunities as those in the wider service. Opportunities for cross-fertilisation should be sought and created.

Supervising the content of work

Even knowledgeable and skilled staff make mistakes and get stuck. Regular supervision of the content of the work is therefore essential for all staff, including those in overall leadership positions. An allowance for this needs to be built into staffing levels. It may be useful to distinguish between supervision of the content of the work (a matter of 'professional supervision') and management of the worker (managerial supervision or 'job consultation' in Manchester). Supervision need not be conducted solely within professions: critical insights can be gained by cross-disciplinary supervision.

Supporting staff

Supervision and management of staff are essential to effectively support them in their work, but other methods are also valuable. Some examples of particular relevance to work with people presenting challenges include:

1 extended team meetings – 'team days' where issues in working with the service users can be examined carefully, and everyone can have a say before an agreement is made on the way forward
2 training and education opportunities, both in areas relevant to behavioural problems and more general issues
3 opportunities for consultation with more experienced and knowledgeable people
4 opportunities for staff to meet with someone independent from their service, to work on their concerns and their emotional reactions to the work
5 team-building activities
6 positive feedback, especially after difficult episodes and successes.

Other ideas will be found in Chapters 3 and 4 on leading and supporting staff.

Ensuring safety

Risk management and physical intervention were mentioned above. Risk management methods can be used to anticipate likely risks, both for service users and staff. Once this is done, means for reducing the likelihood of encountering the risk can be put in place, as well as action plans for those occasions when the risks are met. Increasingly, organisations have their own protocols for this work, and they can be built upon in identifying and managing behavioural risks. Issues to consider might include:

- Self-harm. This includes the ingestion of inedible and toxic substances, plus the secondary consequences of self-harm (for example, dealing with tissue damage).
- Aggression to others:
  - causes, situations and activities presenting high risk
  - procedures and protocols for managing violent situations – when to withdraw, when to intervene, the use of barriers and physical restraint
  - safe practices

- training
- secondary consequences – for example, recovery for staff who have been involved in an incident, dealing with public concerns if incidents happen in public places, protocols for dealing with bites
- vulnerability of others, including other service users, plus issues of incompatibility and grouping.

- Environmental damage. This encompasses hazardous consequences, the use of safe glazing for windows, electrical safety and so on.
- Arrangements for summoning assistance.
- Arrangements for first aid.

Physical intervention is a controversial area, and the reader is referred to the relevant sources (Coates, 1994; Harris *et al.*, 1996; McDonnell and Sturmey, 1993) in order to make informed judgements. As the use of physical restraint is likely to occur in situations when staff are confronted by serious physical aggression, organisations must ensure that safe practices are agreed, followed and monitored. Approaches must be individualised and take place in the context of a wider intervention plan for reducing the frequency and severity of aggression. The Manchester Joint Service has produced a comprehensive policy that could be used as a model.

Constant enquiry

It has been stated above that behavioural challenges can be perplexing and intractable. Considerable progress can be made, but an arrogance about having found the definitive approach must never be allowed to develop. Instead a commitment to constant enquiry is necessary. This means continual review of assumptions, hypotheses, procedures, and practices. Within this style of work, provisional conclusions are drawn; these enable work to continue, and assumptions and hypotheses to be tested. Judgements will have to be made about how long to pursue a method of working or intervention before deciding that it is ineffective or counterproductive.

The staff team needs to work with a true model of 'democratic centralism': there is democracy in the team meeting where approaches can be questioned, assumptions challenged, phenomena reinterpreted, and new approaches proposed. Once the team has arrived at an agreed way forward (best done by a led consensus) then everyone should stick to it until the approach is next reviewed. Within this strategy there can be provision for an emergency review of approaches if they appear to be creating distress or regression.

This approach allows a culture of enquiry which leads to decisions on agreed actions that are themselves subject to the process of enquiry.

Experience in Manchester

The remainder of this chapter will describe the experience in Manchester of establishing what has been called 'clinically managed social care' (not an ideal term, but one that captures at least part of the 'not only but also' thinking presented in the previous section). This experience illustrates many of the issues described above.

Clinically managed social care: origins of the model

The clinically managed model has its origins in work with a young man, whom we will call Paul. He has the condition of autism which, in practical terms, means first and foremost that he finds it particularly difficult to make sense of the world around him. The impairment seems to operate at a fairly fundamental level of information processing, and the result is that the world becomes an unpredictable, frightening place. Social interactions and changes (particularly moving from one place to another) are very stressful. Behaviours of severe social withdrawal, obsessions, repetitive (sometimes self-injurious) acts and destructive outbursts can develop, particularly if little is done to accommodate the person's vulnerabilities (Happé, 1994; Frith, 1989; Williams, 1996). All this was true for Paul.

The first author (MB), in his role as a psychologist, had developed a way of enabling Paul to engage in activities for extended periods of time, as an alternative to the extreme withdrawal and repetitive self-stimulation that he would otherwise engage in almost constantly in his room or in the toilet. This work drew on an educational approach and developmental theory developed by Geoffrey and Bee Bee Waldon in Manchester, although the work with Paul could not be called a pure implementation, influenced as it was by notions from behavioural and environmental psychology. It had not proved possible for Paul's regular staff to work in this way. In early 1991, with the appointment of staff specifically deployed to work with people who presented behavioural challenges, it became possible to sustain and develop what had so far only been exploratory work. Julie Darlington and Alan Lewis not only did this, but also produced impressive evidence for the effectiveness of this way of working, developing the approach into a more comprehensive analysis of Paul's difficulties, and strategies for dealing with them. However, this was only in the context of 24-hour, seven days a week service provision, and the inconsistencies in Paul's care still led to regular outbursts.

A period of upheaval followed in some of Manchester's services, in which both day service and residential staff took industrial action. Following concern about the standards of care for Paul and others expressed by the director and chair of social services and others, an agreement was made with the Central Manchester NHS Trust (this was before the merger of community health services in the city, and three years before the establishment of the Joint Service). This involved a transfer of resources to the Trust which would employ its own staff to support Paul in his own house. However, the house would continue to be part of the network of dispersed housing, which meant that there was no need to establish separate systems for cover, repairs, furnishings and so on. From the outset, the house leader was managed by the social services network manager for the purposes of housekeeping and day-to-day management, but clinically supervised by senior staff in the Trust with knowledge and experience of how to work to reduce behavioural challenges.

From this beginning, the clinically managed houses within the networks developed. At the time of writing there are three, with perhaps two more likely in the near future. The complex needs day service (see Chapter 8) also works within this model.

The house leaders are qualified and experienced learning disability nurses and are known as assistant clinical managers. Within the networks they have equivalent status to the assistant network managers, but are responsible for one house rather than two to three. The original house leader is now the clinical manager who has overall responsibility for the content of 'clinical' work in the three houses. He also has other responsibilities (he is the Joint Service's lead trainer for 'Responding to Aggression and Violence', and 'Physical Intervention'). Consequently, all the staff working in these houses are managed as an integrated team, whether they are employed by social services or the Trust. The houses function as part of the networks; this largely prevents a 'them and us' culture and ensures cross-fertilisation – for example, on standards of care, methods of staff deployment, staff management and so on. Figure 12.2 shows the organisational arrangements.

All the service users had very poor reputation. All but two were engaging in one or more of the following behaviours when the service became clinically managed, and all had histories of at least one of these behaviours:

- assaults on others
- severe withdrawal
- obsessionality that restricted activity and opportunity
- panic reactions
- self-injury
- destruction of environment
- health-threatening behaviour – for example, coprophilia, coprophagia, eating a very restricted diet.

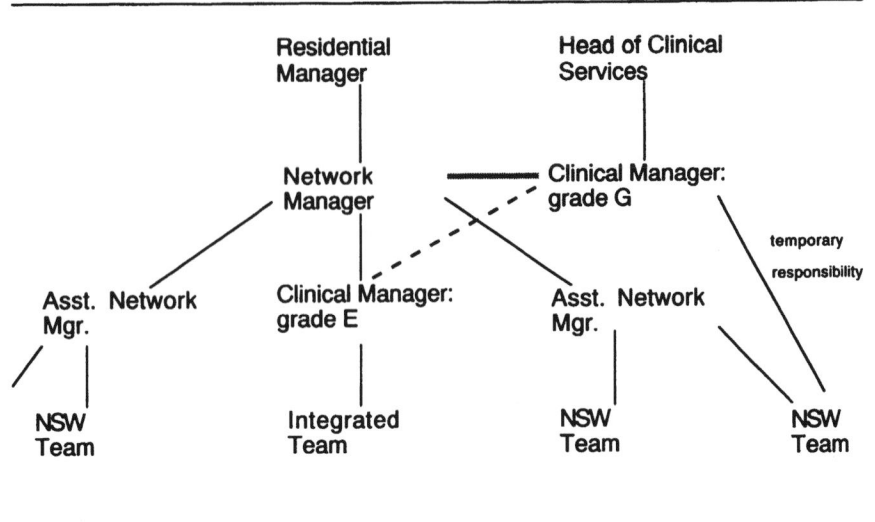

Figure 12.2   Organisational structure for the clinically managed houses

Table 12.1 shows other characteristics of the people served.

The development of these services can be regarded as a 'replication', in which the characteristics of each service and its users differed, but the general approach remained the same. Table 12.2 presents the service developments as a 'replication study'.

Table 12.3 shows the interventions used in each setting, and the evaluation data available to the service in order to assess the effectiveness of the service. Table 12.4 presents global ratings of progress for each service user, based on a consensus of staff involved. Such ratings are, of course, open to bias, but the results are validated in the statements of relatives of service users, as well as by independent observers, such as purchasers.

However, a detailed evaluation is to some extent beside the point: as Bob Dylan put it, 'You don't need a weatherman to know which way the wind blows'. Some changes are very obvious, and sensitive instruments are not needed to reliably detect them. The results from this development do not allow us to identify which interventions, if any, were particularly critical. However, the different start dates for each part of the service, as well as different staffing, do allow some confidence that the 'not only but also'

Table 12.1 Characteristics of the people served in the clinically managed houses and the complex needs day service

House/day service	Service user characteristics
House 1	1 Autism 2 Autism and (?) obsessive compulsive disorder
House 2	1 High-functioning autism (Asperger's syndrome) 2 Autism 3 Severe learning disability and intractable epilepsy
House 3	1 Autism* 2 Severe learning disability
Day service	1 Autism 2 Autism* 3 Autism 4 Autism

* Same person.

Table 12.2 The development as a replication study

Setting	No. of people	Implementation date	Present staffing Qual/ Unqual.	
House 1	2	April 1992	1	5.5
House 2	3	Jan 1993	1	7.5
House 3	(3) → 2	Nov. 1994	2	5.75
Day service	4	Sept. 1994	1	2.6

Setting	Clinical leadership at all times in start up?	Team recruited first?	Rating of ease of implementation (rank)
House 1	√	√	1
House 2	×	×	4
House 3	×	×	3
Day service	√	√	2

Table 12.3   Interventions used in each setting

Setting	Main interventions	Main sources of evaluation data
House 1	• Positive programming • Structured day • Clear boundaries • Specific guidelines and programmes • Person-specific communication styles • Physical intervention • Drug treatment for obsessional behaviour	*Quantitative*: programmes, incidents and activities *Qualitative*: 1 interviews with stakeholders; observation; analysis of documentation.* 2 self-report by one service user
House 2	• Structured day • Clear boundaries • Negotiated activity • Positive programming • Specific guidelines and programmes, including person-specific communication styles • Physical intervention (restraint for one service user)	*Quantitative*: data on programmes and incidents. *Qualitative*: self-report diary and letters from one service user
House 3	• Positive programming • Clear boundaries • Specific guidelines and programmes • Person-specific communication styles • Physical intervention (physical barrier or restraint for one service user)	*Quantitative*: data on incidents.
Day service	• Structured day • Structured activities/positive programming • Structured teaching • Person-specific communication styles • Clear boundaries	*Quantitative*: incidents, behaviour/mood state ratings, activity log. *Qualitative*: service user-specific objectives, detailed review by purchaser

* In addition, all houses are subject to checks on standards of care.

Table 12.4 Global results

Setting	Outcomes to date
House 1	7
	6 → 4
House 2	6
	6
	5
House 3	7*
	5
Day service	6
	7*
	6
	6

Key to global ratings:
7   Dramatically better
6   Greatly improved
5   Some improvement
4   About the same
3   Worse
2   Much worse
1   Dramatically worse

model of 'clinically managed social care' was responsible for considerable improvements in people's quality of life and a reduction in behavioural problems.

Challenging behaviour has been considerably reduced, but not eliminated. The people concerned have many years' practice in using such behaviours: the service has been successful in reducing their need to resort to these repertoires so often. The service cannot, and should not, control all sources of uncertainty and stress: people have to deal with these things, and it would appear that they are becoming more successful in doing this.

To make this service possible, the following support structures have been put in place:

1   clinical line of supervision.
2   location within the mainstream service, for cover, routine management, care audit and so on.

3   training
4   clinical 'on call' arrangement, for 24-hour response, seven days a week, which gives staff confidence
5   additional professional input (chiefly speech and language therapy, psychology, and psychiatry)
6   a culture of problem analysis and solution which draws on the charts and other recording that staff keep and which helps them know that, although progress is slow, the direction is still being maintained.

With several service users, the style of work is not dissimilar from that carried out by some specialist providers: what is different here is that, in Manchester, it is part of the general learning disability service. Challenging behaviour services can become isolated from other provision very easily: different rules can begin to apply, and the result can be very damaging. Moreover, the service is available to people in the community to which they belong, although unfortunately it is not yet available to everyone who needs it.

Perhaps some clues about the important features of these services can be found in these comments by Paul's parents, recorded in interview with Caroline Malone:

> We were so impressed with the way they worked; you could see right from the start. We were always kept informed of what was actually going on.

> ... the way they started to work with him was very good, from getting up in the morning the day was planned right through every minute of the day.

> ... I think programmes had been done in the past for Paul but had never been carried through. ... a very structured approach for Paul, and consistency, which we've said for years we've always known how people should work with him.

> I think they did so well. It took them a long time to get some of the steps forward, but they got there.

While we have been fortunate in working with some exceptionally gifted and committed staff, the general approach could be used anywhere. It can be difficult to implement effective provision in a complex organisational context, but the overall Joint Service model does support the local interleaving of social support and clinical knowledge and guidance.

Acknowledgement

This work relied on the commitment and skill of others, especially Julie Darlington, Lisa Jones, Hamish Kemp, John O'Leary, Alan Lewis, Andrew Pope, Alison Wren, the network managers involved and, of course, the many highly motivated front-line staff. We are grateful to Paul's parents for their permission for us to use their quotations, and for their agreement and encouragement and to write about the work with Paul.

References and resources

Beange, H. and Bauman, A. (1990), 'Health care for the developmentally disabled. Is it necessary?' in W.I. Fraser (ed.), *Key Issues in Mental Retardation Research*, London: Routledge.

Coates, A. (ed.) (1994), *Physical Intervention*, Whalley: Regional Advisory Group on Learning Disability Services.

Doyal, L. and Gough, I. (1984), 'A theory of human needs', *Critical Social Policy*, 4, 6–38.

Doyal, L. and Gough, I. (1991), *A Theory of Human Need*, Basingtoke: Macmillan.

Emerson, E. (1996), *Challenging Behaviour: Analysis and Intervention in People with Learning Difficulties*, Cambridge: Cambridge University Press.

Frith, U. (1989), *Autism: Explaining the Enigma*, Oxford: Blackwell.

Happé, F. (1994), *Autism: An Introduction to Psychological Theory*, London: UCL Press.

Harris, J., Allen, D., Cornick, M., Jefferson, A. and Mills, R. (1996), *A Policy Framework to Guide the Use of Physical Interventions (Restraint) with Adults and Children with Learning Disability and/or Autism*, Clevedon: British Institute of Learning Disability.

Kiernan, C. and Qureshi, H. (1993), 'Challenging behaviour' in C. Kiernan (ed.), *Research to Practice? Implications of Research on the Challenging Behaviour of People with Learning Disability*, Clevedon: BILD Publications.

Lovett, H. (1996), *Learning to Listen: Positive Approaches and People with Difficult Behaviour*, Baltimore: Paul H. Brookes.

McDonnell, A. and Sturmey, P. (1993), 'Managing violent and aggressive behaviour: towards better practice' in R.S.P. Jones and C.B. Eayrs (eds), *Challenging Behaviour and Intellectual Disability: A Psychological Perspective*, Clevedon: British Institute of Learning Disability.

McGee, J.J., Menolascino, F., Hobbs, D. and Menousek, P.E. (1987), *Gentle Teaching: A Non-aversive Approach to Helping Persons with Mental Retardation*, New York: Human Sciences Press.

The Appendix lists some helpful strategies.

Manchester Learning Disability Services (1997), *Responding to Aggression and Violence: Including Policy on the Use of Physical Intervention*, Manchester: Joint Learning Disability Service.

Williams, D. (1996), *Autism: An Inside-out Approach*, London: Jessica Kingsley.

13 Confidence in the community: partnerships to improve the public safety of people with learning disabilities

Dave Crier, Mike Petrou and Mark Burton

Introduction

Modern service development has emphasised the right of people with learning disabilities to be present in, and make full use of, their community. In supporting this, services are learning to become less intrusive and less visible. In the main, this has desirable effects: people are less obviously marked out as 'different', and services are less likely to obstruct natural relationships. However, as with any gain, there can be risks.

Our society is increasingly polarised. For example, Hutton (1993) has described the 'third-third-third society', with the labour force split into the one-third in full-time, pensionable employment, one-third in insecure employment and the highly marginalised remaining third which includes the 10 per cent of the labour force that is unemployed and the 20 per cent working for less than 60 per cent of average earnings. Learning-disabled people will often share neighbourhoods with people who are themselves living in poverty, with little to hope for and subject to the stresses of life in an increasingly competitive society. In such circumstances, social solidarity breaks down; there is alienation and crime. For people who are already vulnerable, there can be additional risks of being victimised.

The case should not be overstated; there is still a huge reservoir of goodwill, mutual respect and support, but this has been weakened by the economic and social policies of the last 18 years. The question, then, is how we can reduce the risk of learning-disabled people becoming victims of crime, without reducing their opportunity to share in community life.

Key issues and guidance

Improving the safety of learning-disabled people in public requires four sets of actions.

1   Assess and manage risk.
2   Enhance community supports.
3   Gain the cooperation of agencies concerned with law enforcement and public safety.
4   Enhance the knowledge and skills of learning-disabled people.

To rely on any one of these in isolation would be insufficient.

Assessing and managing risk

Knowing and understanding the likely risks means that action can be taken to minimise both the likelihood of encountering them and their negative consequences. The extent to which a risk can be prevented will vary, depending on its particular characteristics. There are various approaches to risk assessment and management, but all have in common some variant of the following process.

1   Identify positive reasons for engaging in the particular activity – or being in a particular place, meeting particular people etc and so on.
2   Identify what could go wrong (the risks), together with their likelihood and their seriousness.
3   Form a judgement of the balance between the positive and negative outcomes – relative likelihood, seriousness of the negative outcomes, potential benefits of the positive ones.
4   For each risk, identify ways of reducing the likelihood of encountering the risks; for each method, make a judgement of its feasibility, appropriateness, and likely effectiveness (primary prevention).
5   For each risk, identify ways of reducing the impact of each risk should it be encountered (secondary prevention); review each as for primary prevention.
6   Decide the following:
    a)   Should the activity be pursued?
         If *yes*:
    b)   What methods of primary and secondary prevention can be put in place?
         If *none*:

c) What alternative way is there to realise the positive consequences that would have followed from the activity?

Enhancing community supports

It seems strange that we should have to work to build a community which both includes and supports its more disabled members, but that is unfortunately still the case. The key focus here is on creating and using opportunities for enhancing the mutual support and civic responsibility of communities. This might take a variety of forms, and examples might include:

● taking the opportunity to meet neighbours of group homes
● developing and supporting citizen advocacy, leisure volunteers or similar schemes
● engaging in planning ventures with housing providers to create neighbourhoods where people will be visible when they come and go
● encouraging membership of community-based organisations on the part of learning-disabled people and their allies.

A framework for this work of 'increasing the competence of the community' can be found in Burton and Kagan (1995).

Gaining the cooperation of agencies concerned with law enforcement and public safety

The police and other agencies concerned with law enforcement, crime prevention and public safety can play an important role in preventing crime against people with learning disabilities. However, this is unlikely to happen unless service providers take responsibility for taking the first steps, and encouraging their involvement. Some examples of useful strategies include:

● assisting households with learning-disabled members to join local Neighbourhood Watch schemes
● obtaining advice from crime prevention officers
● making contact with the community police officer – for example, to introduce people who are particularly vulnerable in the local community because of their lifestyle
● attending locality-based police liaison committees where these exist
● establishing joint projects that include police, fire service and others.

Enhancing the knowledge and skills of learning-disabled people

Finally, it is important to work with learning-disabled people themselves to enhance understanding of both potential dangers and safe actions and behaviours. This work uses the same methods of skills teaching that should be well known throughout learning disability provision. As well as enhancing skills it is worth taking simple precautions, such as ensuring that people carry a contact card should there be an untoward incident.

Areas of learning might include:

- how to avoid danger
- how to get out of potentially difficult situations
- how to summon help.

Examples from Manchester

The two examples that follow combine the strategies of involving other agencies and enhancing the skills of people with learning disabilities.

Telesafe

Telesafe is a partnership between the Joint Learning Disability Service and Greater Manchester Police. The partnership was initiated in 1992 following concern locally and nationally about the growing number of reported crimes perpetrated against learning-disabled people.

The initial stage was to identify what crimes were most likely to be committed against the learning-disabled population. A survey, carried out in the city to establish this, revealed that they were theft, fraud and assault. The next stage was to explore several methods of equipping people with knowledge and skills to make them less vulnerable. Video was chosen, chiefly because it was assumed that information presented in this form would be easier to retain than that which relied on the verbal medium. A video production company was engaged, and the social services department agreed to fund the project.

Initially two videos were made in collaboration with some service users and a local drama group. They covered two common scenarios:

- collecting money from the post office and being robbed by a group of youths

- people living in a shared house being harassed by local children.

The videos are designed for repeated viewing by the service users and staff. Repetition is important in aiding retention, and the medium of television is one that is familiar and liked by most service users for whom some degree of independent living is a reality. The video shows inappropriate and appropriate responses to the threats in each scenario. A trademark of the Telesafe style is a red cross which appears across the screen for the inappropriate response, and a green tick which appears with the correct action. The emphasis is on preventive measures to reduce the risk of becoming a victim of crime. Subsequent videos will focus on what to do if one becomes a victim of crime.

The partnership with the police has raised awareness of the interests of learning-disabled people (as has other work on the service's policy on abuse) on the part of the police, and highlighted issues of crime protection and safety within the Joint Service.

In 1996 Bradford Social Services Department and West Yorkshire Police joined the partnership. A different video production company is working with the newly named Telesafe Consortium to produce a video focusing on the problems of bogus callers, distraction burglaries and the dangers encountered on public transport. A publishing and conference promotion company will be marketing the video, and there will be a national conference to launch Telesafe II.

Crucial Crew

Crucial Crew is an event that aims to teach people in an interesting and realistic way how to avoid becoming victims of crime, and to know what action to take in a variety of emergency situations. It is led by Greater Manchester Police and was well established locally in targeting school children in the 9 to 11 age range. The police and the other emergency and utility services involved in Crucial Crew worked with the Joint Service to adapt the event for adults with learning disabilities. The first event for learning-disabled adults took place in June 1996.

Crucial Crew involves the police, emergency services and other organisations working together to create realistic theatrical settings. Each organisation has its own scenario, and those attending the event split up into groups of five or six. Each group visits the different scenarios in order to have the opportunity to experience an emergency or dangerous situation. Since its inception in 1991, there have been a number of reported successes where children have been able to use their Crucial Crew knowledge in real-life situations. Through participation in the event, lives and property have been saved by young people who have put into practice the information given to them at Crucial Crew.

It took a great deal of work to adapt the Crucial Crew concept for learning-disabled adults. A steering group was established, consisting of staff from the dispersed supported housing networks, a community police officer and a representative from People First (a self-advocacy organisation). This group looked at the existing scenarios in order to decide which would be most appropriate to the lifestyle of adults with learning disabilities. It also attended a Crucial Crew event, which gave them a fuller understanding of the methods involved and an idea of the different aspects that would need adaptation. Most of the scenarios were appropriate, but those by Greater Manchester Police and those on Safety in the Community and Safety in the Home needed changes.

The existing police scenario was replaced by a new one in which a service user witnessed a robbery: the main learning points were to not intervene and to be able to give a description to the police. The Safety in the Home and Safety in the Community scenarios required less extensive changes.

Decisions were made about the structure of the day itself and how long each scenario would last. Each scenario was eight minutes long, which seemed brief, but this provided a highly focused period of learning.

A briefing session was held for representatives of each organisation on how they would interact and put information over to participants.

A group of service users from the south of the city was invited to attend the event, all of whom were individually supported by staff from the networks or the community teams. These support workers attended the Crucial Crew on the morning of the event: this was to give them an idea of what to expect and would enable them to support the service users more effectively.

The event itself worked very well: participants gave very positive feedback on local radio and in the press. The working group produced a booklet and video to enable support staff to continue and follow up the work commenced on the Crucial Crew day.

Further events are scheduled on an annual basis.

Conclusion

This chapter identified the vulnerability of learning-disabled people to crime and exploitation – a phenomenon that is still underrecognised. A framework was offered for enhancing the public safety of people with learning disabilities. Two examples, each from Manchester, 'Telesafe' and 'Crucial

Crew' were described, both of which combine two strands in this frame-work: building collaboration among service and public safety organisa-tions; and enhancing the skills of learning-disabled people.

References and resources

Burton, M. and Kagan, C.M. (1995), 'Increasing the competence of the community' in *Social Skills for People with Learning Disabilities: A Social Capability Approach*, London: Chapman and Hall.

Hutton, W. (1993), 'Three thirds Britain' in S. Wilks (ed.), *Talking About Tomorrow: A New Radical Politics*, London: Pluto Press.

Kemshall, H. and Pritchard, J. (1996), *Good Practice in Risk Management*, London: Jessica Kingsley.

Telesafe (Video) (1995) Halifax: Hebden Lidsay.

Williams, C. (1993), 'Vulnerable victims? A current awareness of the victimisation of people with learning disabilities', *Disability, Handicap and Society* 8 (2).

14 Using video for service development

Nigel Hoar and Mark Burton

Introduction

We live in a televisual age. For better or worse, television and video provide a common reference point or shared source of experience. Televisual sources grab attention in ways that the written word or speech alone cannot.

In the last ten years, portable camcorders have become available to a wide cross-section of the population, allowing social events to be experienced once through participation (or through the viewfinder!) and then again on the screen. The representation of events on the screen both reproduces and redefines their reality.

With such a potentially powerful medium available, it is worth exploring its use in representing and developing the experience of learning-disabled people and the services that support them.

Video has a particular relevance to people with learning disabilities and their services. Intellectually disabled people face barriers in accessing information which is important to them, and which will often be in a format that they cannot easily understand. Very few service users can read well, but nearly all watch television. Many people have other sensory and cognitive disadvantages including hearing loss, poor sight or problems in understanding speech. Video can be particularly helpful in supporting the communication process.

Video can also be useful for staff and others. Sometimes it is important that care and support is given in a particular way. While written procedures and guidelines can be helpful, they rely on staff reading and internalising text. A video can demonstrate the appropriate methods, catching the nuances of interaction that the written word is less able to describe.

A more traditional use is in the analysis of behaviour–environment relationships. While often valuable, this more technical augmentation of professional skills will not be described here.

Key issues and practical guidance

Purposes

It is important to be clear about the purpose of producing video. This will determine the scope of the production and its degree of sophistication: for some purposes 'home-video' style productions will be adequate. For others, semi- or fully professional production will be necessary.

Purposes include:

- documenting people's everyday life and experience as a 'portfolio' for planning meetings
- documenting service developments for funders, other parts of the service or training purposes
- documenting appropriate (and inappropriate) practices for purposes of staff support and training
- assisting learning-disabled people to develop skills and experience in production and presentation
- assisting self-advocacy and the projection of the user voice.

Resources

Resources required will depend to some extent on the type and volume of video production to be undertaken. It will be worth identifying a 'video coordinator'. The person is likely to have (or will soon acquire) knowledge of video production techniques. A minimum requirement would be knowledge of how to use a camcorder and home video recorder to carry out edits using the pause and record buttons. The role is initially likely to be an additional responsibility.

The coordinator would liaise with the people who had commissioned the video (for example, the service user and carers) to agree its objectives. It may be useful for someone (for example, a key worker) to devote time to researching particular aspects of the video content, such as collating old photographs in chronological order. It is difficult to give guidance on time requirements as they depend so much on the nature of the videos to be produced.

Consumables are the tapes required and the production of still prints if a cover is to be made for the videotape box. Money should be budgeted for general repairs of the equipment and the replacement of video heads. It is advisable to use the best quality tape – unfortunately the most expensive! Video tape comes in a variety of formats, usually VHS. However, camcorders usually use either 8 mm video tape or VHS-C (the C standing for compact, which means that, via an adapter they can be played back through a standard video player without the need to connect up cables to the recorder). There is also SVHS, SVHS-C and Hi 8, superior tape which produces a much clearer picture and is particularly useful as the editing process degrades picture quality. Recently, digital video camcorders have been manufactured that produce almost broadcast quality picture and sound for a fraction of the cost. With the use of an appropriate computer for editing there is virtually no loss of quality.

The basic list of equipment needed is as follows:

- 8 mm or VHS-C camcorder
- video recorder with pause/record facility
- television to use as a monitor
- sturdy fluid head tripod.

Access to a video/film makers' cooperative or similar resource is useful for learning skills and accessing equipment.

Production and editing

Video production is time-consuming. Besides the time needed to film there is a need to reconnoitre the film location and plan the filming. Editing is often a lengthy process depending on the type of finished product desired and whether graphics, photos, and so on are to be included. For the videos produced for the Joint Service, an average of two hours' editing has been needed for every minute seen in the final production.

It is important to have aims and objectives for the video and an idea of the target audience before starting to film. The format can be discussed and set out in 'storyboard' form (see Figure 14.1). This is basically a small pictorial representation of each shot and any notes or any preplanned dialogue. Any directional prompt or particular shot (for example, a wide shot) should be noted below the picture.

Where service users are involved they should be allowed to have maximum editorial control. This can be achieved by letting the service user watch the playback of the video and decide which footage to include and

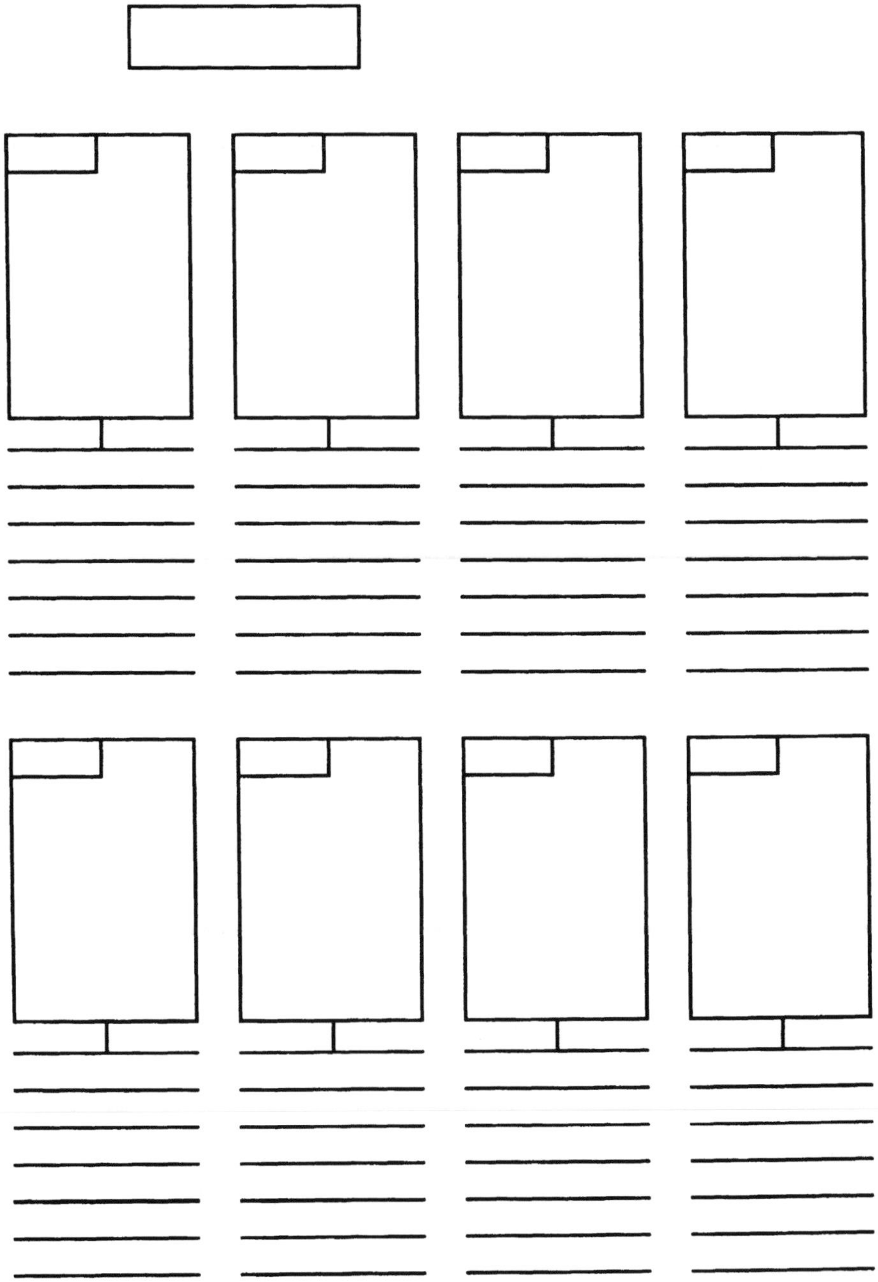

Figure 14.1   Storyboard for video production

exclude. If the person is unable to do this then it would be desirable for someone who is close to them to take on this responsibility.

Dissemination

The way a video is distributed will also depend on the purpose for which it was made. For some purposes, such as describing how to work effectively with a particular person, only one copy will be made. Other purposes – such as documenting a person's experiences and preferences – might require a small number of copies (say, for the person, their house team and their family). Finally, some purposes call for larger-scale production, marketing and distribution (as in the Telesafe project described in Chapter 13 or in the case of the 'Listen to Me' conference described below).

Permissions, confidentiality and copyright

Video involves making a record of people's actions and circumstances. Everyone has the right to be consulted about this, and permission will be required to share this record with others. Video records of individuals are regarded as equivalent to written case files in health and social services and are therefore subject to the same requirements of confidentiality and security of storage. However, with consent, this information can be divulged and can also be shared for the legitimate purposes of providing a service. Not all video recording would be regarded in these terms (for example, a film of a football match would not). The principles governing the video recording of learning-disabled people are no different from those for anyone else in their public and private lives, but the issues of consent are likely to be more complex.

The form used in Manchester for consent to the use of photographic and video materials is reproduced in Figure 14.2.

Examples from Manchester

Shared planning: portfolios

Videos have been produced, showing people's past and present experiences and future plans, and showing what is important in their life. This format is understood by many service users and forms a basis for further work in person-centred planning (see Chapter 17). For people unable or unwilling to attend their planning meeting, it may be possible for them to be represented

---

LEARNING DISABILITY SERVICES IN MANCHESTER

CONSENT FOR THE USE OF PHOTOGRAPHIC AND VIDEO MATERIALS

1 Name and address of person to be photographed:

   Name:
   Address:

2 Name and designation of photographer:

   Name:
   Designation:

3 Purpose for which photographic material is to be used:

4 I agree that the person named above may take still or moving photographs of me. It has been explained to me how the photographs are to be used.

   Signature:
   Witnessed by:
   Name:
   Designation:
   Date:

or

5 Acting on behalf of   I agree that photographs may be taken for the purposes stated above.

   Signature:
   Name:
   Relationship:
   Address:
   Date:

Figure 14.2   Form for consent to the use of photographic and video materials

by their video. For people with sensory impairments, subtitles can be added, and signs and symbols added where these are used. Particular attention is paid to the soundtrack – for example, by using the person's favourite music. If English is not the first language of the target audience, then it may be worth dubbing the video into the appropriate language.

These videos – which have been a source of great pride for some of those involved – form a permanent record of the person's life and help them in the process of obtaining more control over it. The video also conveys subtle information about the person – for example, how they demonstrate excitement and pleasure and their various skills (for example, fine or gross motor skills, domestic and social skills).

Watching the video, preferably with the service user present, can be included in the induction of new staff. This helps staff obtain an authentic picture of the person they will be supporting, which adds to information in the person's personal records. It can be supplemented by the staff member's growing experience and the information conveyed by colleagues. It can also help prevent the development of myths and false assumptions about the person that can so easily enter the culture of staff teams.

User involvement: 'Listen to Me'

Chapter 16 on user involvement, describes the 'Listen to Me' conference. A video record made of this conference showed both the process of supporting people to express their views, some of the views stated, the responses of management panel members and people's evaluations of the conference. A copy of the video was supplied to each person who attended the conference, and it was played at the recall conference held later at which panel members reported back on actions they had taken on the issues raised.

Recording a service development: 'The allotment'

A garden project was set up by one of the Joint Service's dispersed supported housing networks. Service users and staff have worked together to create a productive and aesthetic environment on a site where other gardening enthusiasts also rent allotments.

In a video made of the project, a service user interviewed participants and other people at the allotments including neighbouring gardeners and delivery men. Other service users were involved in the filming and the editing.

This video both presented the project to other parts of the service and involved people in the recording of it, giving them great pride in their involvement.

Resources

Access to Health Records Act (1990), London: HMSO.

Department of Health (1995), *Code of Practice on Openness in the NHS*, London: Department of Health.

Wayne, M. (1997), *Theorising Video Practice*, London: Lawrence and Wishart.
Examines implications of, and possibilities for, radical grassroots video production.

Books on home video production are readily available, and are constantly being updated as newer camcorders and recorders bcome available. The magazine *Camcorder User and Desktop Video* has proved very useful as it covers subjects such as basic editing and gives information and prices of various pieces of equipment.

For those in the North West, the Workers Film Association in Manchester is a very helpful community-based resource, running a number of different courses from beginner to semi-professional standard. They are able to hire out equipment and editing facilities at competitive rates.

Part IV

Safeguarding Quality

Introduction

The final three chapters are all, in various ways, about safeguarding the quality of the service, which ultimately is about the quality of service users' experience.

In Chapter 15 Mark Burton and Helen Sanderson provide an analysis of quality and its promotion that emphasises a participative, multiple safeguards approach. They illustrate this by drawing on the considerable amount of work on securing quality that is being carried out in the Joint Service.

Karen Goodman reviews ways of empowering the users, or customers, of services to influence their design and operation in Chapter 16 'Service User Involvement'.

Finally, individual planning has long been seen as a desirable component of effective learning disability services. In Chapter 17 Helen Sanderson identifies some of the problems of the traditional methods and draws on recent developments in Manchester and elsewhere to present a more imaginative and empowering approach to planning with people.

15 Quality

Mark Burton and Helen Sanderson
with contributions by Iain Larkin, Dave Ruane,
Allen Briscoe and Karen Goodman

Introduction

Quality is particularly important in learning disability services. In any organisation that provides a service to people, quality is closely bound up with the reason for the organisation's existence. However, in learning disability services, a population with little power is served by organisations with considerable relative power over their day-to-day experience and life courses. This imbalance means that quality can be vulnerable to influences that have little to do with the interests of people who use the service. There is no particular conspiracy here, but rather a set of forces or tendencies that, together, can submerge user interests and quality beneath a fog of apparently rational reasons and excuses. Some examples of these systemic threats to quality include:

- financial pressures
- interests of staff, managers, families, other organisations
- drift from high standards over time
- societal position of disabled people: relatively low status and priority.

Indicative of this vulnerability is the poor record of learning disability services in the past. The scandals of the 1960s should be well known, but these are only the tip of the iceberg in the systematic second-rate opportunities historically offered to people with intellectual disabilities. Recurrent themes have been identified by writers such as Wolfensberger in the response by society and its services to severely disabled people. These include:

- segregation from the ordinary life of those in the mainstream of society
- being grouped together with others on the basis of disability, dependency, or stigma
- isolation
- loneliness
- having a negative reputation
- being treated in ways that are dehumanising
- poverty
- a lack of power, choice, autonomy, self determination
- limited opportunities or help to grow, or develop
- insufficient help in getting important things done
- threats to health or personal integrity
- vulnerability to exploitation or ill treatment
- an identity that is dominated by the role of 'client' (Burton and Kagan, 1995).

Partly in response to this situation, the philosophical change of the 1970s and 1980s led to more dispersed services. These present a different challenge if quality is to be safeguarded. Service provision in private spaces can make monitoring more difficult – although it is worth stating that the authors have witnessed the worst provision in institutional settings and the best in ordinary houses, and research findings also bear this out. Moreover, when living in close proximity to ordinary members of the community, vulnerable people and their care can be more visible and open to concerned questioning and representation than in segregated facilities.

As services became more local and dispersed through the 1980s and 1990s there was a parallel emergence of consumerism in health and welfare provision, together with an explicit rhetoric of quality in both managerial discourse and that surrounding the promotion and implementation of the quasi-market in health and social care and support.

It is to this constellation of factors (systemic vulnerability of service users and the quality of their provision; explicit philosophies of care and dispersed, less visible provision; the emergence of a legitimated discourse of quality in these sectors) that approaches to the promotion and safeguarding of quality must respond.

Key issues

What is quality?

It is important to base our understanding of quality of service on its contribution to its users' quality of life. Unless we do this, we risk promoting
changes that, while promoting *organisational* effectiveness, have little relevance to the people who rely on the service. However, we also need to go
beyond a mere equation of quality of service with quality of life since
quality of life depends on a variety of factors which includes, but goes
beyond, services. To the extent that quality of life does depend on the
service, it is important to understand the characteristics of services (and
organisations generally) that promote and support high-quality experiences
for service users.

Quality of service, then, can be understood in terms of a relationship
between the quality of life of the people who use the service and the quality
of the supports which the service provides to enable the experiences that
contribute to a good quality of life. Figure 15.1 illustrates this.

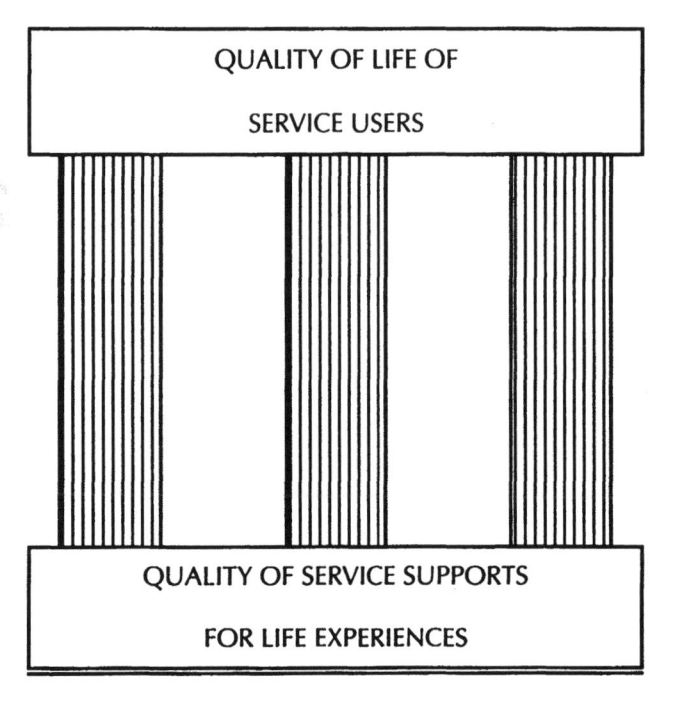

Figure 15.1   Relationship between quality of life and quality of service

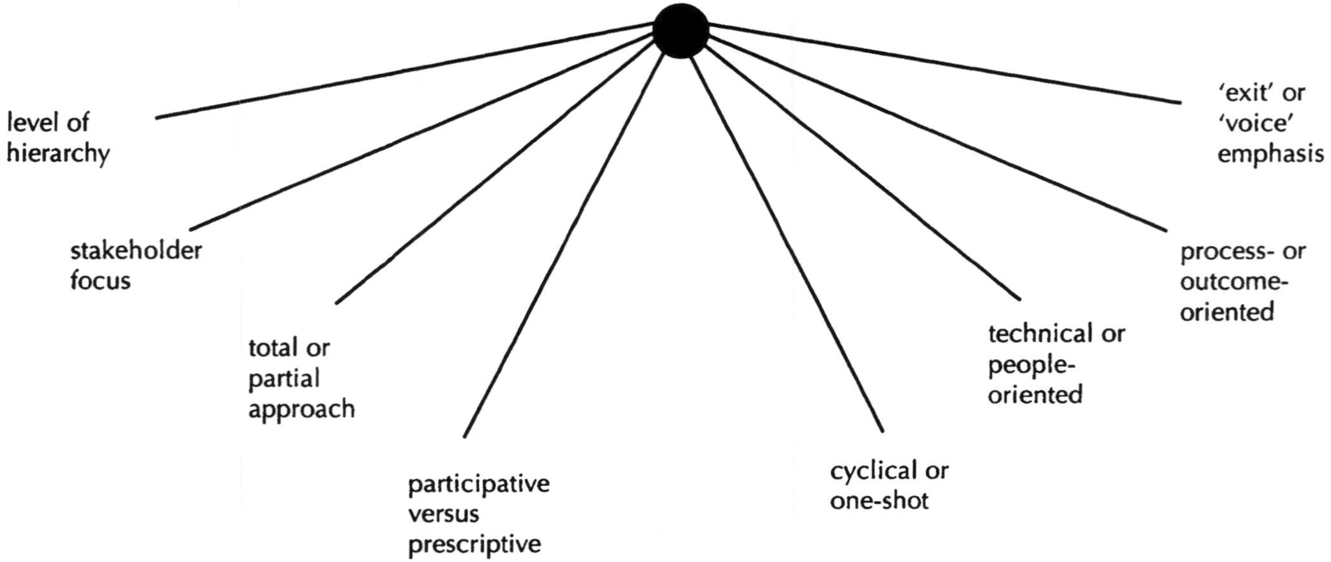

Figure 15.2 Classification of approaches to quality

level of
hierarchy

stakeholder
focus

total or
partial
approach

participative
versus
prescriptive

cyclical or
one-shot

technical or
people-
oriented

process- or
outcome-
oriented

'exit' or
'voice'
emphasis

This way of thinking defines the overall aims and philosophy of the service, which should be explicitly stated – for example, in the form of a 'mission statement and services principles' or 'statement of aims'.

Given the above overall definition, there can still be various frameworks for describing quality and its pursuit. Figure 15.2 shows a classification that might be helpful in understanding the different approaches that have developed and their interrelationships.

Level of hierarchy

Quality can be approached at all levels of the organisation from senior management to front-line staff. In terms of influence on service users' experience of life, it is the front-line staff who have most influence. However, it is worthwhile trying to establish a consistent approach to quality throughout the organisation, and this involves all levels. In a hierarchy, some levels monitor the quality of performance of subordinate levels.

Stakeholder focus

Different strategies emphasise different stakeholders. So a quality strategy that depends on a complaints system emphasises service users, their allies and community members (all of whom might make complaints) and managers (who have to investigate and resolve complaints). A strategy based on contracts monitoring will emphasise the role of purchasers in quality assurance.

Total or partial approach

Some approaches to quality attempt to develop a total culture of quality, with all the processes, procedures and structures of the organisation oriented towards the pursuit of high-quality outcomes (for example, as in Total Quality Management). Other approaches pick one or more key elements in the service as the focus of quality strategies.

Participative versus prescriptive

Some approaches to quality – for example, those based on standardised production procedures – are highly prescriptive, with the organisation only having to translate the approach into their own context. At the other extreme, it is possible for the staff of an organisation to create a unique approach to quality from the 'bottom up'. In the latter case there may be a greater chance of ownership of the agreed approach, but there is also a high risk of the approach losing momentum once the initial enthusiasm of invention and development has worn off. Moreover, there is a possibility of repeating others' mistakes. In practice most approaches will involve the participation of the workforce and other stakeholders, within a framework prescribed by management or outside bodies (for example, government, purchasers, inspectors).

Cyclical or one-shot

Some quality initiatives involve a once-and-for-all, or one-shot, effort. The replacement of institutions with community living options can be regarded as a large-scale, one-shot quality strategy. More often, the pursuit of quality requires a cyclical process of inquiry and action, leading to closer and closer approximations to quality while circumstances also change. A common fault of failed quality strategies is that this loop is not closed: evaluation and audit does not lead to action, standards are not audited or quality action plans are not implemented.

Technical or people-oriented

Quality can be understood in technical or human terms, or as combining both aspects. Technical aspects of quality include standards, indicators and the technology of measurement in general. Human aspects include qualities such as vision, commitment, leadership and the culture of the service. To focus exclusively on one or the other aspect is likely to lead to an ineffective conception both of quality itself and the ways of achieving it.

Process- or outcome-oriented

Example

A survey was carried out of families whose disabled members were using a new care management service. Their evaluations were extremely positive. On closer examination, the service had made little discernible difference in terms of life experiences (outcomes) available to the disabled family members. The survey had focused almost exclusively on the process of the service, and the time taken by the new care managers plus their respectful attitude to the families (who had had little provision in the past) accounted for the very positive evaluations.

This distinction was discussed above in relation to quality of life – an outcome and a quality of service – which includes process, as well as structure. In assessing quality it is important to be aware of whether process or outcome is being addressed.

'Exit or 'voice' emphasis

Recent policy has emphasised the role of consumer choice and the logic of the market in introducing incentives for high quality in services. To gain an improvement, consumers have to 'exit' from one form of provision and enter another. An alternative approach emphasises the consumers' 'voice' in the political struggle for a better deal. Again, both elements may be important, and an exclusive emphasis on one at the expense of the other can lead not only to an impoverished conception of quality but also to a reduction in the levers available for influencing quality.

Achieving quality

The above classification suggests some important dimensions of an effective quality strategy. Before putting them together, a further issue must be raised: can quality be assured?

A moment's reflection suggests that, in human services, there is always scope for fallibility, confusion and the unexpected. This means that talk of 'quality assurance' which might make sense for a chocolate factory, is overoptimistic and perhaps likely to lead to simplistic strategies. These are unlikely to cope with the variability and richness of the provision of effective services by real organisations to real people living real lives in real communities!

On the assumption that 'what can go wrong often will', a different approach suggests itself – that of 'belt and braces' or of 'multiple safeguards'. No one approach will protect vulnerable people from poor services and the decline of standards, but a combination of approaches operating in different ways, at different levels and with different stakeholders, can reduce the risk and indeed positively promote higher quality.

A 'multiple safeguards approach' then, might include:

- clarity about the purpose and methods of the service
- external inspection and review
- internal setting and monitoring of standards
- robust processes for encouraging good practice and discouraging poor practice

- positive encouragement of complaints, together with means to take corrective action
- monitoring the overall pattern of service development
- the measurement of outcomes
- a culture of accountability
- a continuing dialogue with service users and their allies, based on a recognition of the need to listen and work together for improvements.

Practical guidance

The foregoing review of issues suggests a general approach to the pursuit of quality, and the resources listed at the end of this chapter give more guidance. In addition, it is worth emphasising the following points.

Clarify expectations

As indicated above, the pursuit of quality needs to rest on a clear statement of what the service understands by quality and how it will attempt to achieve it. A 'mission statement' or similar should be agreed, with consultation from stakeholders (see below). It is essential to find ways of keeping everyone focused on such a basic definition of quality. It is also vital that it is presented and re-presented in a fresh, imaginative (but not gimmicky or trite) way, so that all actions – including decisions, policies, training, and practices – can be related to it. It may be worth considering tactics such as:

- printing it on the headed paper the service uses
- putting it on all policies, internal communications, individual planning forms, team brief, and so on
- actively referring to it in management meetings, service planning and staff supervision
- presenting reports under headings derived from the service principles.

Involve stakeholders

Quality typically involves change, and people affected by change need to feel involved in it. It involves commitment: it is difficult to impose quality without ownership by those affected. It is therefore important to identify the stakeholders in any service.

Exercise: involving stakeholders

A community team has a catchment population of about 100 000 in a small northern town. It serves people with learning disabilities, most of whom live with their families, but some of whom are in a variety of supported housing and small residential services provided by the social services and by the independent sector. The team comprises social workers/care managers, community nurses, a psychologist, speech and language therapist and two occupational therapists. The post of physiotherapist is vacant. The team is coordinated by a NHS manager, with some delegated authority for the social services staff. A separate manager is responsible for a team of peripatetic care staff, who work from the same building.

Try to identify the stakeholders for this service.

The stakeholders in the above exercise might include:

- learning-disabled people with learning disabilities and their representatives (for example, self-advocacy groups)
- their families
- staff working in the team
- the manager and his or her manager
- the peripatetic care staff working closely with the team, and their manager
- independent sector providers
- those purchasing the services provided by the team
- trade union representatives
- client advocacy organisations (for example, MENCAP, VIA, if local groups exist).

The above is not an exhaustive list; we might also include local community interests, other referring agencies – such as GPs, day services, schools, and so on – but not everyone can be involved in everything. Different types of service will have different profiles of stakeholders.

It will be important to identify the nature of the stake, which the above interests have in the service: what do they stand to gain or lose as a result of improvements in quality? Are they likely to have different emphases in thinking about quality? What would be considered as enhancing quality?

Some will want to play a central role, while others will just want to be kept informed.

In implementing quality initiatives, it is helpful for the jobs to be shared, so that the different stakeholders have responsibility for events. This also has the added advantage of people working together and better understanding one another's perspectives. Quality should not be the sole responsibility of management or of a quality function in the organisation, although it is valuable to have someone whose remit is to lead and coordinate the work of others in this sphere of concern. Similarly, quality cannot be achieved just on the basis of a contractual arrangement: purchasers are only one of several types of stakeholder (and their activity should also be subject to scrutiny in terms of quality!).

Create a culture where quality really matters

If quality is to be seriously pursued, then leaders in the service must emphasise (and theorise) quality at all times. While attending to the other organisational tasks in the service, quality must remain central, with all decisions taken in relation to the 'So what?' question:

How will this affect the quality of experience of those who rely on the service?

Building a culture that hinges around quality means:

1   continuing to pursue quality as you do other things, and
2   publicising quality strategies, initiatives, and achievements.

Pursue quality as you do other things

How can the day-to-day management of a service be underpinned by the pursuit of quality? Quality is not an 'optional extra' for human services, but a basic requirement. While external safeguards and the internal review of services are important, in the last analysis they can only be effective if the service can make principled changes – that is, if it is run in an organised way so that the myriad of day-to-day decisions can be informed by an understanding of their likely effects on users' quality of experience.

Such changes will have to be made at all levels of the service organisation, from the level of strategic/senior management up to that of the management of individual programmes of care.

As it happens, there are already many structures, processes and activities that are sites for the decisions that determine the quality of the service. These can be used as the basis for managing for quality.

Commitment to quality

The management of human services must be understood to be more than a technical affair. It involves harnessing the disciplines of management – strategy and organisation, managing people, analysing information – to the lives and experiences of those who have to depend on services. To do it well requires a commitment to real improvement in the conditions of people with major disabilities. Such commitment must be the basis for all decisions made in the management process, if quality is to be achieved.

Managing in three directions

The effective management of the service for quality requires managers to face three ways (see Figure 15.3). As the figure shows, for each domain, a series of activities, tasks, processes and structures can be identified, which, taken together, comprise management.

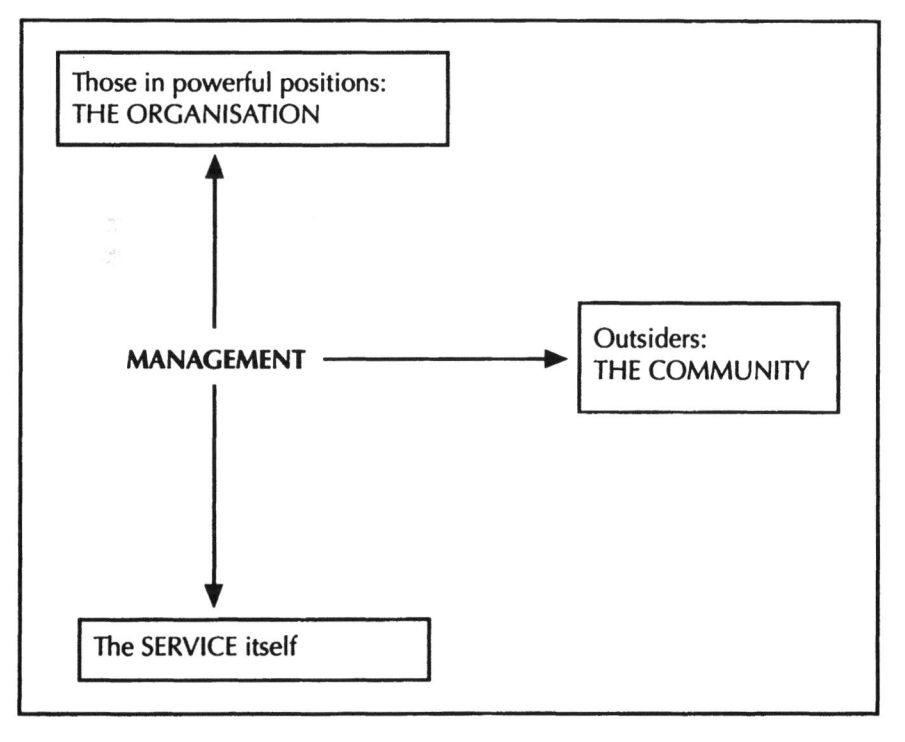

Figure 15.3   Managing in three directions

Transactions with those in powerful positions in the organisation

---

Example

How could each of these be handled in ways that create greater quality of experience for service users, both now and in the future?

- visits from authority members
- meetings with Senior Managers
- input to organisation's planning process/cycle
- appraisal by superior manager
- monitoring by the organisation
- linkage with management supports (for example, finance, personnel, planning, information specialists)
- input to budgetary process
- crisis meetings.

Transactions with outsiders from the community

Example

Each of these can be handled in ways that enhance, or detract from, users' quality of experience:

- receiving visitors
- shopping
- dealing with tradespeople
- accompanying consumers in a variety of community activities
- relationships with immediate neighbours
- involvement in community organisations:

    - as a service
    - as an individual with an interest

- involvement with other services and service-type organisations (for example, the police, GP, dentist, schools, youth organisations)
- any obvious community events and structures that can form the basis for additional transactions with the service (for example, carnivals, church fêtes, harvest festivals and so on).

Transactions with the service itself

Example

Each of these can be a great opportunity to obtain a little more quality:

- staff supervision and appraisal
- team meetings, retreats, review days
- expenditure decisions
- recruitment and selection (all elements)
- documentation of work carried out
- policy formulation
- training
- organisation of staff deployment and work allocation
- report preparation
- monitoring of the service – informal/formal
- production of written guidelines
- disciplinary action
- negotiation with unions
- interservice meetings.

Each of the above topics can be regarded as an opportunity for managers to improve quality – either of people's experiences or of the service supports for a good quality of life.

Example: staff deployment

Services often squander their most valuable resources – the time of their staff. Many use only the most primitive mechanisms for planning their deployment. As a result, there can be too few staff at critical times, and unoccupied staff at other times.

If staff deployment stems from an analysis of what the service is specifically trying to achieve for and with its users, then managers can more rationally allocate this scarce resource so that it is used effectively and efficiently.

The precise mechanisms will depend on the particular service. Whether staff are deployed in a way that supports quality can be assessed through asking these questions:

- Is the staffing level the same at all times or does it vary according to need and activity?

- Are staff ever on duty with nothing to do (for example, when clients are at day services and there are no team meetings, training, individual-focused meetings, or administrative or organisational tasks scheduled)?
- Do staff always know what is expected of them?
- Are service users stuck in their setting for long, unbroken periods of time?

The above examples illustrate the availability of many potential 'levers' that managers can pull to promote quality. In effect, every action of a manager should be based on the conscious pursuit of quality: a failure to do so, or a view of management as disconnected from quality issues, is usually indicative of poor management and poor services.

Without a strong commitment to quality and the assumption of responsibility for quality on the part of managers then quality is unlikely to materialise in the lives of those who depend on the service.

Publicising quality strategies, initiatives, and achievements

A further aspect of creating a culture of quality is the permeating of the service with an awareness and understanding of quality, and what those in the service are doing to enhance it. The following strategies can be helpful:

- publicise quality initiatives taking place within the service
- offer briefing for staff and managers on quality and strategies which provide safeguards
- market the service in terms of its quality characteristics rather than on merely financial or technical aspects
- emphasise quality in internal and external statements and documentation
- seek external feedback, help, and validation for what you are working on.

Use quantitative and qualitative information

Information can come in various forms, and each has its advantages and disadvantages. One distinction is between qualitative and quantitative – primarily about whether the information is in the form of numbers (*quantitative*) or in the form of verbal accounts, prose, poetry, mime, pictures, or some other non-numerical form (*qualitative*). In addition, however, quantitative methods tend to be associated with approaches which divide subject-matter into small parts, while qualitative methods tend to involve the description of the subject as a whole. Quantitative approaches also tend to be associated with the pursuit of objectivity though the non-involvement or distance of the investigator from the people whose service is studied. Qualitative approaches, on the other hand, tend to emphasise the pursuit of understanding through engagement or close contact with the people concerned with the service.

It is increasingly being recognised that both quantitative and qualitative methods are legitimate – the choice of one or the other depends upon the question being answered by information gathering.

Quantitative methods	Qualitative methods
● Provide more manageable information to analyse and compare, but limit information to a restricted set of predetermined categories.	● Produce rich and detailed information allowing study of issues in depth without the need for predetermined categories for analysis.
● Attempt to break down complexity into parts.	● Attempt to present complexity for what it is.
● Are easily summarised and presented but summary data may be misleading unless interpreted with caution.	● Are relatively difficult to summarise and present findings, but information is often in the forms of people's own words which can speak for themselves if allowed to.

A balanced approach would therefore combine qualitative and quantitative techniques, using the strengths of each. Generally speaking, the larger the object of study (say, for example, all the services in a city) the more it will be necessary to rely on quantitative techniques, while the smaller the object of study (for example, a single one service programme) the more it will be feasible and essential to emphasise qualitative approaches.

It should be stressed that both quantitative and qualitative methods can be concerned with quality.

Closing the loop: quality improvement as change management

It is not enough to talk about quality, measure it and identify areas for improvement. The 'loop' must be closed with action to secure improvements. If quality is to be improved, then actions will have to be identified, and those with responsibilities for these actions monitored and held accountable for carrying them out.

A familiar cycle can be identified, and all parts are essential (see Figure 15.4).

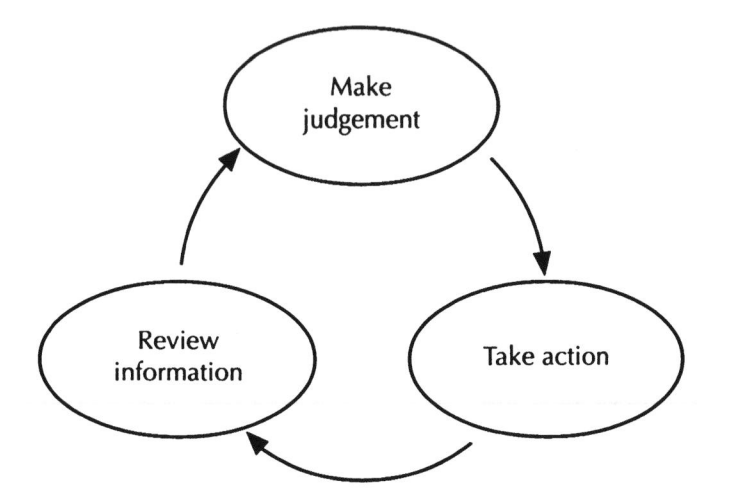

Figure 15.4   The 'loop' of information, judgement and action in managing for quality

Examples from Manchester

In Manchester the Joint Service's approaches to quality were initially founded on an audit developed in response to a crisis, followed by a focus on standards, policies and procedures then evolving into a 'multiple safeguards approach'. The following diverse initiatives will be described.

- Standards and audit
- Multiple safeguards and the quality action group
- Good practice – *Service Principles into Action*
- 'Putting quality into management'
- PATH
- Consumer conference
- Professional supervision
- Stakeholder involvement
- Quality projects:

- Outcomes
- Complaints
- Good practice by fieldworkers when working within the network houses project
- Implementing planning study.

Standards and audit

One of the first formal moves towards monitoring quality commenced before the establishment of the city-wide Joint Service as a result of a crisis in a hostel where people were living in unacceptable conditions. Following the investigation into this, the director of social services demanded that measures were taken to ensure that this could not be repeated. In response, managers identified areas which needed to be monitored on a regular basis. Initially this happened without a set of clear standards as a reference point in deciding whether conditions were acceptable.

To establish standards, a methodology developed within nursing was borrowed, and managers trained in it, which enabled them to understand the concept of standards and how to devise them. This was to be linked to an auditing process – that is, the monitoring method by which regular achievement, or failure to meet those standards, was measured.

Those first standards principally related to management support strategies such as job consultation (supervision) and team meetings, in an attempt to ensure that personal support was being guaranteed to each staff member.

The second step was for each network to begin producing its own standards. Within a six-month period each of the networks had devised a plethora of operational standards covering many operational and support issues: it quickly became clear that this was a road to hundreds of standards, policies and procedures, ensuing mountains of paperwork and cumbersome and time-consuming audits.

Instead, a group representative of the service came together with the joint managers to look at the mission statement and each of the main areas for which the service was responsible. These were the beginning of the 'service principles', based around the accomplishment framework which are used in the service today. For each service principle, the group identified key indicators – three or four for each principle – and assigned someone to coordinate a representative group of staff to develop the standards and audit for that area. The coordinators for each standard were given training in setting standards and audit, and a timescale was established for drafting the standard and audit, consulting on it, then being ratified by the senior managers. This was an ambitious project. It was a total approach, as each of the service's main areas of responsibility were addressed, but focused on key elements of the important processes and outcomes. It was participative in that there was an opportunity for people at all levels within the organisation to be consulted and involved rather than 'buy in' existing packages of standards which staff did not 'own'. It suffered from loss of momentum after the initial enthusiasm as there was no one at that time who had a particular responsibility for quality issues within the service. As a result of that process, the networks developed 26 standards and developed two main audits – the revised house visits and a monthly organisational audit which gave information about training, sickness and so on. This was developed into what is now known as the 'house visit' audit – a 'yes/no' audit used by assistant network managers (ANMs) on a quarterly basis. This was a simple form which indicated each of the standards, against which it could be stated whether that standard had been met, and if not why not. Over time, and because of a need to computerise the format to enable easy access to the information, the standards themselves became a series of questions on given areas of support which could be answered by a simple yes or no. As the consultation process around this form progressed, sub-questions were added.

The network inspection form, as it became known, was completed quarterly by managers visiting houses unannounced. The audit is divided into sections on the condition of the house inside and out, and staff record-keeping at the house. The audits were put on to a database so that graphs and feedback could be given to managers and staff on a regular basis and actions could be set from the information produced. The audit provided a useful starting point for thinking about quality and shifting the culture of the residential services towards an acceptance that we needed to systematically develop and monitor the quality of the service. It was recognised that this audit only focused on 'technical' information rather than being people-oriented or addressing quality of life issues and therefore other initiatives were required to achieve a balanced approach.

The benefit of the system, which was perhaps unforeseen, was that it gave teams a simple quarterly task list of work which needed to be done. Although much of this was routine, such as basic housework, much of it also related to the decorative state and safety aspects of the houses and was used to correct many deficiencies. By creating a systematic approach to carrying out of both minor and major repairs, it ensured that the condition of the housing environment improved. It was the managers' own tool, and having committed themselves to it, they were also committed to the improvements it required.

Multiple safeguards and the quality action group

These experiences made it clear that, whilst the well worn cliché rightly states that 'quality is everyone's business', in practice this needed to be guided by people who take a specific lead in this area. In the move to the Joint Service one of the Joint Service managers was mandated to develop quality, and a representative group was formed to work with him to tackle these issues. Initially, the group focused on standards, policies and procedures and audit issues, but over the months it became clear that a much broader emphasis was required to develop multiple strategies.

The group spent time reflecting on the nature of quality. Following the 'Roads to Quality' approach (Burton, 1993), the purpose of the service (as identified by the mission statement) was examined. As a result, one of the group's early initiatives was to consult people about developing and re-writing the services mission statement and service principles. These then began to be used throughout the service as part of each quality initiative rather than just appearing in the business plan. The initial approach to developing multiple safeguards involved:

- continuing the development and review of standards, policies and procedures
- developing a good practice guide to go beyond merely describing minimally acceptable standards
- looking at quality in management with a 'putting quality into management' initiative
- orchestrating the use of the PATH planning process for each team to set their objectives for the year based on what takes the service closer to the service principles and mission statement
- working with People First to organise a consumer conference to hear what the people who use the service think about it and want changed
- regular analysis of complaints and recommendations for action.

Good practice – *Service Principles into Action*

Working to define the minimum standards for the service occupied much of the group's early work. It was recognised that, while it is very important that staff know the standards below which the service must not slip, they also need a shared understanding of what good practice is to work towards. It cannot be assumed that the mission statement and service principles are interpreted and put into practice in the same way by different staff. For example, like many services, Manchester has seen abuses of the principle of supporting people to develop choice, and a clear understanding of the issues involved in balancing informed choice, safety, and personal growth has not always been present. As a result, the ideology of 'choice' has on occasion shaded into neglect.

Developing an understanding of what the service principles look like in action took place in two parts. The first was for network and community team staff to identify and share what they considered to be good practice – giving very practical, day-to-day examples. This was collated and put under the relevant service principle identifying what the good practice was for each principle and also the converse – the practices to avoid. This explicitly spelt out what the service is aspiring to, using staff's own words and examples, and which practices were to be avoided. The resulting guide, *Service Principles into Action*, is used on all induction and values-based training or 'service philosophy' courses. Teams also refer to it in evaluating their own practices. The guide cannot remain static, but is subject to regular review. Manchester People First is helping to review it and ensure that it also reflects what service users want. For example, the support that service users want in planning for themselves as described in the book *Our Plan for Planning* written by People First in Manchester, and Liverpool has been added to the guide.

The service principles also refer to staff being recruited, supported and developed to enable them to meet the needs of service users, ensuring that staff are informed and involved in decision-making. The second development, *Service Principles into Action for Staff*, involved looking at the support which staff and managers receive and identifying what is good practice and poor practice. This was completed by asking all staff to write down a specific example of a time when they felt very supported and a time when they did not. These examples were then listed together and emerging themes identified which could be divided into management–staff issues, and staff–staff issues. As a result, two guides to best practice have been produced covering each area.

'Putting quality into management'

The 'Putting quality into management' project running from the year 1997/98 acknowledges that quality initiatives and safeguards need to take place at all levels in the service and not just focus on hands-on workers. The initiative builds on the work done under the heading 'service principles into action' and focuses on three main areas:

- identifying management skills and getting feedback
- providing managers with training – 'managing for quality'

- increasing the time managers spend directly with staff and service users.

The themes that emerged under 'service principles into action – for managers' were as follows:

1 being available and actively listening
2 valuing others and considering their feelings
3 giving positive feedback and constructive criticism
4 being a reliable leader
5 being informed, sharing information and consulting with staff
6 regular, fair, constructive job consultations and team meetings.

The guide that articulates good and poor practice under each of these headings is being used as the reference point for an 'upwards appraisal' system for all managers in the service. This will combine feedback from staff, feedback from the manager's manager and a self-assessment to identify an action plan for each manager. Implementation began with the five Joint Service managers, and will be cascaded throughout the service.

PATH

An organisational climate questionnaire completed by staff in the Joint Service indicated that many staff wanted to make more of a contribution to the development of the service. One way to move towards this would be to develop the business plan 'bottom up' rather than have it written by managers and then consulted on. PATH – a graphic planning process developed by O'Brien, Forrest and Pearpoint, initially as a form of person-centred planning – was used as a way to approach this. The process can also be used for team and organisational planning. The network managers, the training action group, and shared planning development group had all successfully used it as a process for planning their next year's goals. The process works by having the group reflect on and visualise desirable futures for people with learning disabilities. These may never be completely achievable, but they serve to set the direction and guide the rest of the process. When this has taken place, the next step is to agree specific practical and possible goals to move towards the vision. The remaining steps involve identifying what the situation is like now, who else needs to be involved, what the group will need in order to stay on track and what needs to happen in eight months, four months and two months. The process ends with people making a commitment to the first steps that they will need to achieve in a week to take them towards their goals. It was agreed that each community learning disability team, the network managers, Joint Service managers, training action group, shared planning development group and the quality action group would each spend a day working with facilitators to create their own PATH. Each group looked at the service mission statement and service principles and worked out what they would

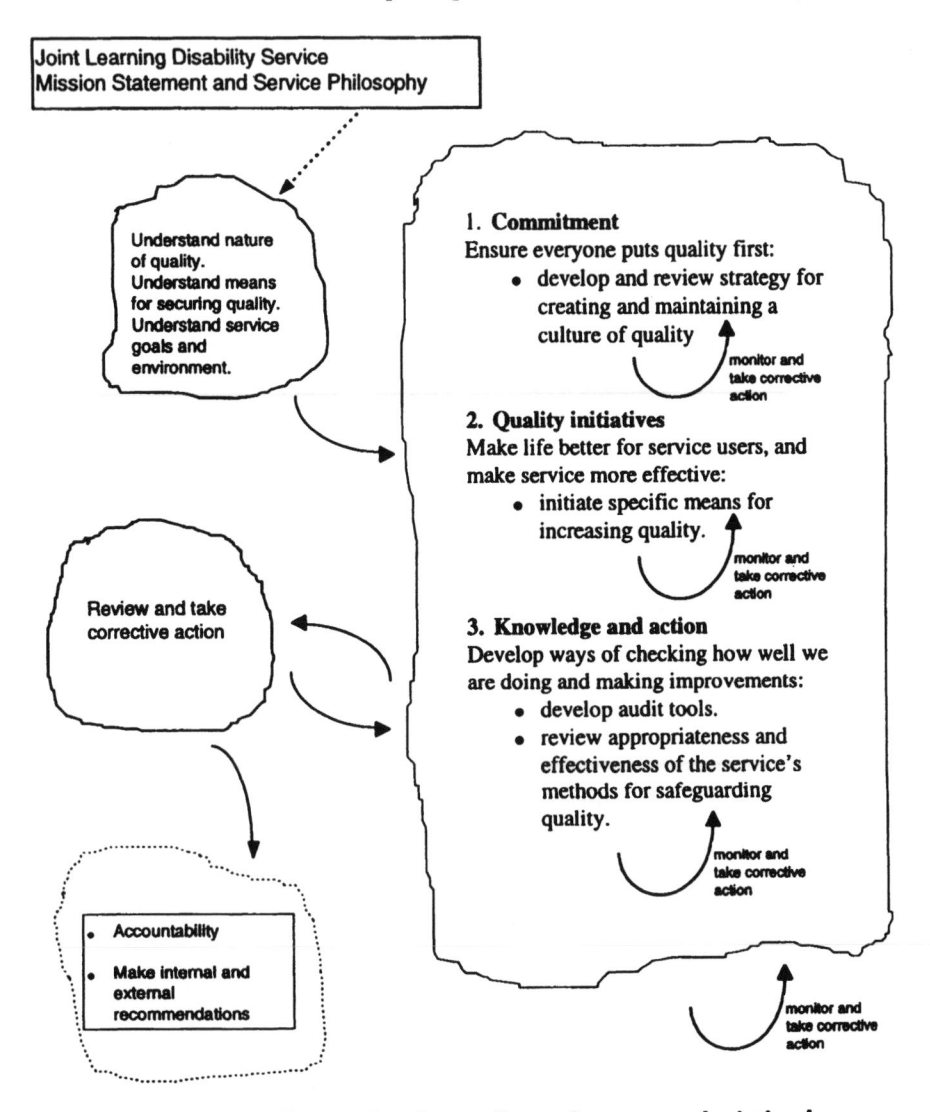

Figure 15.5   Holon diagram for the quality action group, depicting key tasks, information flows and linkages

really look like if realised. These ideas, together with the results of a consultation with service users, parents and carers, formed the framework from which goals were suggested. Finally, specific goals were chosen and prioritised for the team to work on in order to take them closer to that ideal, with a clear understanding of who would do what by when, who outside of the team needed to be involved and how they would support each other in the process. Two representatives for each PATH came together with the Joint Service managers to look at issues that had been raised by PATH that were outside of the control of the teams and should be addressed at service level, and also to look at how PATH would be supported and evaluated by the service. At the end of the process each team had their own coloured, laminated PATH describing the goals which they were working on, a copy of the whole service PATH which summarised the goals which each different part of the service was working towards and a 'brochure' of all the different PATHs, so that they could see in detail who was working on what goal.

In the course of the quality action group PATH, a 'holon' (Checkland and Scholes, 1990) was made, which diagramatically identifies the function and tasks of the quality action group (see Figure 15.5).

Consumer conference

In keeping with the emphasis on strengthening the voice of service users, a major customer conference, entitled 'Listen to Me' was held in late 1996. This is described in Chapter 16.

Professional supervision

All professional staff within the service receive regular supervision from a more experienced colleague from within their profession. There is an agreed protocol for this, and an agreed boundary with the line management function (exercised through regular 'job consultation'). This content-focused input is seen as a key safeguard in ensuring that staff remain focused on user outcomes and use the most appropriate methods available to achieve them.

Stakeholder involvement

The importance of involving stakeholders was identified above. As an example of this in the Manchester Joint Service, Allen Briscoe, the manager of the short-term support service, contributed the following section about developing links and improving communication with families and carers of adults who use the short-term support service.

Manchester's short-term support service began operating as a city-wide service during 1992, having previously been managed as part of several networks which provided mostly long-term supported housing.

The movement from a service that was managed from several locations (and in different ways) to one in which it was managed centrally had several implications, the principal one being, perhaps, the creation of a network of houses spread over a large area, which would rely even more on good and effective communication with the people who use the service.

Supporting approximately 140 families and carers across five sites, using 14 beds (plus two for emergencies) and meeting individual needs relied upon organisation. Giving the individual families and carers, as well as the individuals who directly use the service, access to information, decisions, developments and a voice to talk about the service they received, needed something extra for it to be meaningful. This part of the work concerns the ongoing struggle to create a proper dialogue between service provider and service user – one in which both sides have the opportunity to have their say and know that each other's problems, concerns and worries (as well as the many positive outcomes) are shared and understood.

Although the service is restricted to the resources available, better communication and understanding of needs/desires/hopes of all stakeholders should lead to a more imaginative use of resources, and therefore a better service.

Regular coffee mornings helped. The opportunity to come and share views with staff and other carers with food thrown in was a good incentive. However, it didn't cater for carers who work in the daytime, and other evening sessions had to be arranged.

The development of the short-term support service quality action group was another step forward. It consisted of a parental representative from each property having regular (six-weekly) meetings with the network manager to discuss aspects, concerns and developments within the service. The parental representative was also given the opportunity to help with the quarterly monitoring of the properties. Spot checks and visits to properties are an essential and ongoing part of the management process in ensuring a quality service, but it was decided to carry out a three-monthly comprehensive check on aspects of the service – for example, checks on cleanliness, food availability, medication records, the functioning of smoke alarms and so on. It was therefore useful to include parents in this process, and their comments led to direct action. For example, one parent complained about an overgrown tree at one of the houses. The team immediately hired a skip and spent a morning pruning and cutting. Although we believe that examples like this helped develop relationships and trust, the process still failed to reach all parents and carers. If a parent didn't meet or contact the QAG representative, were they being represented? We decided to develop in several ways.

First, we produced our own newsletter to families. *Time Out* first appeared in August 1996, and will be published twice yearly. Its aims are to keep parents/carers and service users informed of what is going on in our service, but also to involve them in that process. Copies were sent to every family, as well as to other professionals within the service.

Second, we decided to look at developing a representative group for each property, to include the carers who are involved in meeting with us. Two parents from our property in Chorlton responded to our appeal, and have met regularly since July 1996. This will be repeated at other properties during 1997, with the overall aim of having four or five carers or service users who meet regularly at each property and then send a representative to the main QAG.

As a management team, we also meet regularly for team-building sessions. We periodically invite parental representatives to these sessions, again increasing the voice of the paying customer!

In line with this greater accountability, we are also publishing a yearly report in February of each year, outlining basic details, facts, figures and so on of our service for the preceding year. This gives direct information on how well we managed our service and what we were able to offer during the year. It also points out the number of complaints that we received and how we resolved them. However, the key point behind the facts and figures is one of explaining 'why' certain things happened and the pressures which influence our resources and management.

For example, during 1996 one of our properties was closed, due to the wider financial problems faced by the city council. We responded to this by offering all of the families respite at our other four properties and were able to manage the situation, despite the stresses and strains put on to the families and our service. The yearly report gave us the opportunity to further explain the 'why, what, how' as well as our future and current property development plans.

Trying to find better ways of accounting for our service and of informing people of our future aims and intentions, also provided the incentive to keep the momentum of development going. This can only be good for all concerned.

Even with our long-term difficulty, property developments, having to account and inform families of our efforts meant that we couldn't drift into apathy. During 1996 plans were revisited to change properties and to increase our downstairs 'adapted bed' resources. Monies were promised, plans adapted, reports written, but then, as a result of budgetary pressure, funds were reallocated elsewhere and progress was not forthcoming. Having to admit this in newsletters, yearly reports and at QAG meetings, keeps the profile high! Happily, we have responded to changing needs and resources with fresh proposals which have been provisionally accepted, and we offer a more positive outlook for 1997.

We also made contact with other local authorities, and began 'networking', sharing ideas and making contacts. During 1996 we visited Bolton, Stockport and Oldham short-term support services and were able to see the work of other services at first hand. Ultimately this can only benefit our service, and hopefully others.

In conclusion, therefore 'good communication' can only work if it is actually meaningful and responsive. This means that the service can reward itself by saying what it does well, and can produce newsletters, yearly reports and so on to substantiate this. However, it is equally important to admit failures, to listen and act upon complaints quickly and with an open mind, and to account for our actions.

During 1996, when a newspaper article appeared in a local newspaper relating a family's concerns about a 'problem' at one of our houses, a letter was sent to all families, on the same day, by the head of service explaining that the article actually related to an issue which had occurred in 1994 and had been investigated.

It is only by working in partnership with families and people who use our service that trust and communication develop effectively.

Quality projects

The quality action group is supported by two part-time quality and service development officers who coordinate and work on the projects initiated by the group. In addition to these, they work on various 'spot projects' identified by the service. These may be short investigations or longer-term analyses. Examples of these follow.

Outcomes

Field services, such as care management, social work, and health professional inputs, assess need, deliver and arrange service supports and interventions, and monitor client well-being and services provided. They are a cornerstone of community care provision for people with significant disabilities. Most similar services now record some data on the volume and cost of their activity, but little progress has been made in developing methods for either monitoring outcomes at service level or measuring the outcomes produced. Key difficulties facing outcome measurement in field services include:

- the heterogeneity of service users, their needs, and therefore the desirable outcomes – even within specific client groups such as 'people with learning disabilities'
- the historical emphasis on activity or other process measures in such services
- the insensitivity of many global measures of quality of life or adaptive functioning to positive improvement in key domains
- problems of validity and reliability, especially outside a research context
- professional resistance and potential disagreement regarding the appropriate specification of outcomes.

Goal Attainment Scaling (GAS) (see, for example, Kiresuk, *et al.*, 1994) is one approach with potential to overcome these difficulties, and the Joint Learning Disability Service is currently piloting GAS as a means of monitoring outcomes, on a sample basis across its four community learning disability teams. Preliminary work in one locality had previously indicated the feasibility of specifying intended outcomes and scaling their attainment.

The project has:

- prepared a manual for goal specification and scaling
- developed a model for workplace coaching of staff using the approach
- set goals with 10 people, consecutively referred to each of the four teams.

Initial findings on implementation of GAS suggest:

1 the need for a higher profile launch and briefing for a full-scale project
2 the acceptability of the method to families
3 the acceptability of the method to staff, once explained
4 the feasibility of appropriately scaling all types of goals – staff could easily predict the expected level of outcome but needed help in defining the other levels on the five-point scale: the coaching arrangement to iron out conceptual difficulties in goal setting and scaling was valuable here
5 some difficulty in sharing goals with users and carers in a minority of cases (for example, where suspected abuse is being investigated)
6 initial difficulties with scaling assessment work (including community

care assessments), which can be resolved with redefinition in terms of user outcomes ('why assess?') – part of the cultural shift from a focus on process to a more outcome-focused service

7   underrepresentation of work (in the pilot) by professions, with a slower turnover of episodes of care and support (for example, speech and language therapy, physiotherapy)

8   the need for redrafting of some parts of the manual, which although oriented to community care had been based on the therapeutically-oriented North American models.

This work, which continues, has formed the basis for a successful research grant application to the Department of Health to extend and evaluate the approach in the Joint Service's four community learning disability teams.

Complaints

One way for the service to learn more about its impact is through the complaints that it receives. An analysis of complaints received by the service indicated that very few service users were making them. One of the quality development officers reviewed options for making the system more accessible to learning-disabled people. This is described in Chapter 16.

Good practice by fieldworkers when working within the network houses project

This project was established to identify examples of good practice as viewed by fieldworkers (that is, CLDT staff), residential staff, managers and service users. The study concluded that the most successful interventions were carried out by fieldworkers using a facilitative style and working with teams who were committed to the service users, where there was high morale and good communication. Interventions were more likely to have a lasting effect on the service user's life where the team and management were stable and where CLDT staff consulted with, and involved, service users, staff and line managers. A self-audit checklist was devised, to help fieldworkers assess how effectively they are working to secure cooperation with their work.

Implementing planning study

This study worked, over a period of 18 months, with two service users who have profound and multiple disabilities and the staff team and manager who support them. The project developed the use of Essential Lifestyle

Planning and, later, PATH and identified with the team how these planning styles could be put into practice and affect how staff worked on a day-to-day basis (see the staff deployment example on p. 237). The team investigated how they could ensure that the activities and routines identified through Essential Lifestyle Planning took place, how they could record and consistently respond to the service users' non-verbal communications and how they could identify and develop the relationships of service users. As the whole service moves towards using Essential Lifestyle Planning, these strategies will be taught to teams to help them find ways of making sure that people have 'living' plans rather than ones that remain in filing cabinets.

Summary: multiple safeguards in Manchester

The quality action group is working to develop and expand this interlocking range of safeguards and service developments to support a high-quality service:

- **External inspection and review.** The social services purchasers have developed a method of quality assessment which they use, on a sample basis, with people living in network houses.
- **Internal setting and monitoring of standards.** This has been completed for the networks and is in process for community teams.
- **PATHs, and the quality projects.** All of these are 'backed' by job consultation and professional supervision.
- **Positive encouragement of complaints.** A complaints survey has been carried out and consumer conferences are held.
- **Measurement of outcomes.** An outcome study was established to identify how outcomes could be measured in practice.
- **A continuing dialogue with service users and their allies.** A quality action group for parents and carers has been formed to develop the quality of the short-term support services.

For the future, the emphasis will be on consolidating these diverse approaches and integrating them within a coherent whole so that they mutually support one another.

References and resources

References

Burton, M. and Kagan, C.M (1995), *Social Skills for People with Learning Disabilities: A Social Capability Approach*, London: Chapman and Hall, Chapter 1.
Checkland, P. and Scholes, J. (1990), *Soft Systems Methodology in Action*, Chichester: Wiley.

Resources

General material on quality and its pursuit

Flood, R.L. (1993), *Beyond TQM*, Chichester: Wiley.

Approaches to quality in health and welfare services

Burton, M. (1993), *Roads to Quality: A Sourcebook for Improving Services to People with Major Disabilities*, Whalley: North Western Regional Advisory Group for Learning Disability Services.
Carter, R.K. (1983), *The Accountable Agency*, Newbury Park and London: Sage.
Independent Development Council for People with Mental Handicap (1986), *Pursuing Quality*, London: IDC.
Kelly, D. and Warr, B. (1992), *Quality Counts: Achieving Quality in Social Care Services*, London: Whiting and Birch/Social Care Association.
Maxwell, R.J. (1984), 'Quality assessment in health', *British Medical Journal*, **288**, 1470–72.
Nocon, A. and Qureshi, H. (1996), *Outcomes of Community Care for Users and Carers: A Social Services Perspective*, Buckingham: Open University Press.
Schalock, R. L. (ed.) (1990), *Quality of Life: Perspectives and Issues*, Washington DC: American Association on Mental Retardation.

Standards, indicators, checklists, measurement

Cresswell, J.W. (1994), *Research Design: Qualitative and Quantitative Approaches*, Thousand Oaks, California: Sage.
Kiresuk, T.J., Smith, A. and Cardillo, J.E. (eds) (1994), *Goal Attainment Scaling: Applications, Theory, and Measurement*, Hove and London: Erlbaum.
Patton, M.Q. (1982) 'Managing management information systems' in *Practical Evaluation*, Beverley Hills CA: Sage, Chapter 9.
Social Audit Resource Packs: from New Economics Foundation, 1st Floor, Vine Court, 112–116, Whitechapel Rd., London, EC1 1JE. Tel: 0171-377 5696.

On stakeholder involvement and other ways of thinking about improving quality

Dluhy, M.L. (1990), *Building Coalitions in the Human Services*, Newbury Park and London: Sage.

Feuerstein, M-T. (1986), *Partners in Evaluation: Evaluating Development and Community Programmes with Participants*, London: Macmillan.

Whyte, W.F. (ed.) (1991), *Participatory Action Research*, Newbury Park and London: Sage.

Professional supervision

The following texts address a nursing audience, but are actually more generally relevant.

Butterworth, T. and Faugier, J. (1992), *Clinical Supervision and Mentorship in Nursing*, London: Chapman and Hall.

Kagan, C. and Evans, J. (1995), *Professional Interpersonal Skills for Nurses*, London: Chapman and Hall, Chapter 13.

16 Service user involvement
Karen Goodman

Introduction

From the late 1970s onwards, customers of services have become increasingly seen as active participants who have a part to play rather then passive recipients of welfare. Gradually, services are becoming aware of their prime accountability to the people they are there to serve. Increasingly, efforts are being made to provide services and increase quality in such a way that people who use services can be seen as partners. In attempting to give a strong voice to their customers, services aspire to develop more democratic, participative methods of inclusion.

There has been a move away from expert analysis towards the involvement of learning-disabled people themselves. Involvement in engineering change within a service goes hand-in-hand with increasing people's confidence, and helping them feel capable and an important part of the whole process. Empowerment of long-disempowered minority groups comes with increasing control over their future.

The 1990 NHS and Community Care Act requires community care planning to be 'marked by collaboration and by the involvement through consultation ... [of] service users'. It states that community care plans must contain details of how to 'involve representatives of service users and their carers in planning care'.

No longer is it just a question of user involvement being a good thing; it is a statutory requirement. Complaints procedures and consultation over community care plans must now be in place. There is a new emphasis on quality assurance and customer involvement. However, this only goes so far: it is one thing to assert the need for user involvement, but another to make it real.

As with criticisms of the limitations when white people carry out research in black communities, so disabled user groups are calling for research to be carried out by themselves, rather than by 'experts'. Within a quality service, customer participation is not seen in isolation – as an end in itself – but as a developmental process which results in improved service delivery.

A lack of guidance on exactly how to involve customers has led some services to implement methods which, in hindsight, have at best been 'token' efforts and, at worst, been confusing, humiliating and wasteful of customers' time. Gaining insight from others' experiences, reflecting on current practice and considering ways to incorporate successful customer involvement are necessary processes being undertaken in many services, including the Manchester Joint Learning Disability Service. This chapter will examine and discuss some current literature, methods, and examples of involvement.

A note on terminology

Various words have been used to identify those who rely on services. I am uncomfortable with all of them. 'Users' has a cold, utilitarian ring. 'Consumers' implies that human services are like the products of commercial enterprise, and falsely likens people who rely on services to the mythical free agents of the capitalist market. 'Customers' similarly implies a commercial transaction, although allied with the slogan 'the customer is always right', it does suggest the need for a rebalancing of power. In the absence of a better term, I use all three, more or less interchangeably.

Key issues: why have customers not been more involved?

Existing arrangements within services for evaluation, management and development are often unhelpful for involving customers with learning disabilities. Many factors operate against their inclusion, both at a personal and service level. Potential challenges for a learning disability service may include:

1 **Limited intellectual capacity.** Customers will have difficulty understanding information and they may not have all the concepts required to process information. Service personnel often use overcomplex language or jargon. A shared language cannot be assumed.

2 **Ensuring full representation.** Customers acting as representatives may not be reflecting the needs of those from further minority groups, particularly people from non-English speaking backgrounds, those using aids for communication, people with sensory disabilities and those with high support needs.

3 **Inclusion of people with multiple handicaps.** Supporters may try to 'read' behaviour or use a proxy. Potential conflicts here include the impartiality of supporters, the availability of independent advocates and accurate representations of view.

4 **Knowing your rights.** For many years learning-disabled people have been denied rights and may be unaware that the service exists for them. Instead, they have tended to be grateful for any service given, and have so established a weak bargaining position within society.

5 **Acknowledgement of the conflicts of interest.** These can exist between the providers of a learning disability service and its users

6 **Practical difficulties in ensuring sufficiently broad and detailed consultation.** It is sometimes important to try to obtain everybody's opinion, while, for other purposes, a representative sample of opinion will be sufficient. The amount of feedback required may differ for, say, consultation on a new policy, whereas detailed one-to-one interviews may be more appropriate for consultation on a new review system. However, the use of multiple methods will often elicit a fuller picture (see Chapter 15).

Examples

1 Notting Hill Housing Trust used a combination of questionnaires and workshops run by an independent advocacy organisation to find out levels of satisfaction with the housing support tenants received.

2 The Minnesota Governors Council on Developmental Disabilities uses six different evaluation instruments to assess housing provision:

- Parents use a normalisation based questionnaire.
- Service personnel carry out visits.
- House groups use a checklist to discuss their facilities and share results with staff.
- Third-party evaluators visit and interview consumers and staff.
- Observations and interviews by parents and others are sought primarily for views about the 'feel' of the house.
- Training exists for consumers and advocates which covers different types of living arrangements and observational skills.

Service providers should clarify the purposes of user involvement, and question and confirm their commitment to it. The following questions may give some insight into current and meaningful future involvement.

- At which level do we currently involve customers?
- Is there an agreed consensus (at senior management level) for involving customers? Is there a 'service commitment'?
- What purpose will customer involvement serve?
- How can customers be assured their input will be valued? What will be done with the information given to us?
- How can we ensure that our service is as welcoming as possible to customers and that it is as easy as possible to include them?
- Has senior management set standards to ensure the above happens consistently? Within the same service there can be both exceptional and poor practice happening.
- Do customers know their rights? Do they have a list of rights? Would they know where to find out about them?
- Is there an acceptable complaints procedure?

Example

In the Manchester Joint Learning Disability Service it was discovered that there was a distinct lack of complaints from service users. Through a consumer focus group, formed to assess the accessibility of the current system, it was found that not only were customers completely unaware of the system, but there was also limited understanding of the concept of complaining.

- Does the service perceive development as ongoing and increasing, or as final? Are there plans to develop customer involvement?
- What quality controls are currently in place across the service?
- What planning or development could customers be involved in?
- If there are current user groups, are they independent? Have they had enough training? Do they have appropriate ongoing support?

Practical guidance

Meetings

Current practices in running services may be challenged by the inclusion of customers in planning and development. Much business is conducted in meetings relying on a high level of verbal understanding, the ability to read and background knowledge. Even with the benefit of years of job experience, similar life experiences and often professional training of three years or more, meetings can be daunting. Without any of the above they can be confusing and intimidating.

Exercise

Consider how you might feel as a user representative of a service (for example, coronary care) having recently been an inpatient within that department.
Suppose you have to:

- use public transport in a strange town, because you are unable to use, or don't have, your own transport
- go into a meeting of doctors and other clinical staff, all of whom know each other, dressed in suits (when you have come in everyday clothing), with bleeps going off periodically
- listen to medical terminology you have never heard of
- look at diagrams you don't understand
- answer questions about changing cardiac care policies.

Meetings can be further disabling in that they often unconsciously use 'service speak' – language that service workers feel comfortable with: 'network houses', 'additional support team', 'mission statements', and 'complex needs' are all terms frequently used in Manchester, yet may have a different or no meaning in other situations.

People need to know formats, conventions and rules (often implicit) of meetings – for example:

- The minutes from the last meeting should be brought with you.
- You ring before the meeting with 'apologies' if you can't go.
- Often an agenda is followed.
- Meetings are not the place for social chat except to fill in a few embar-

rassing first minutes to put people at their ease: if you do speak, you should say something but not too much, and so on.

- Meetings often last between one and two hours. Difficulties arise if you can't tell the time or estimate how much time has passed.
- Reading and writing are often required: nearly everything is written, even if there is the odd picture.

Other barriers include the fact that meetings are usually held during the day – this suits service personnel but can be difficult if you have a job or a regular daytime commitment. Finally, staff typically have cars to get there, but customers have to get the bus.

Questions to ask before deciding on meetings

1 What precisely are you hoping the customers can assist with? e.g.

- providing information?
- stating their views?
- making decisions?
- designing better service responses?
- or is it to raise awareness or just so people feel involved?

2 Is this the most appropriate way of doing this or would a different method be more suitable? For example:

- focus groups
- detailed interviews
- participant observation
- surveys
- shadow meetings and parallel groups
- service user-run evaluations
- service user involvement in staff training
- briefing sessions.

3 Is this group willing to adapt the way it runs meetings?

You've decided on meetings. How can they be more useful?

Preparation It is much easier to become involved when you are clear about the topic, background information, your role, expectations and what has happened as a result of these meetings in the past.

Timing Find out what is the most suitable time for a service user to meet prior to arranging a time with service staff. Are you willing to meet in the evenings or on days off?

Payment Much customer involvement relies on them giving up time on an unpaid basis to help a service develop. Too often people volunteer their time and effort, possibly unsure as to whether it will make any difference. Acknowledging that customers' time should receive payment, as ours does, puts more value on their input and increases commitment from staff to fully consider their role and reasons for inclusion. How many staff would come to a meeting without payment?

Examples

1 A country-wide working party on gender issues paid all its researchers and is now able to calculate costs for future projects.

2 Customers in Manchester have recently been paid as consultants for a few pieces of intensive work in developing shared planning through a research fund.

3 A conference held in Manchester recently paid People First for acting as facilitators.

Training and support for key participants

Examples

1 In Minnesota, USA, customers had five days' training, and technical assistance after this, so that they could carry out monitoring and evaluation.

2 In Washington State, USA, support for involvement in meetings involves reading information, explaining discussions and materials in less complex language.

Using representatives/advocates People First, an international organisation for people with learning disabilities, has developed a number of localised representative groups across the UK. The role of an advocate is immensely valuable, within services, for those with learning disabilities. It is also demanding, as representatives need to feel confident that they have fully understood what has been conveyed by the customer. They also need to feel comfortable in relaying this to management and other stakeholder groups.

Shadow committees   In this format, a group of customers discuss, in a different setting or format, the minutes of a meeting and decide what comments they wish to pass on. It can also help to develop a understanding of the likely agenda issues.

Example

One Manchester district planning group used a shadow committee successfully before the group was disbanded due to a change in joint planning arrangements. Their shadow committee met an hour before the district planning group and then passed information to the meeting.

Twinning   Each customer joining the group is partnered with an existing meeting member who joins them before the meeting, explains the proposed discussions and supports them throughout.

Careful management of documentation   It is worth colour-coding any written materials – for example, the fixed agenda could always be green, the works report could always be pink, and so on.

Keep written information to a minimum; instead, use videos, graphics, pictures, role play, sculpting, photography, verbal repetition and recapitulation of main points.

Documentation is discussed more generally on page 265.

Feedback   Ongoing, clear and explicit feedback of the outcome is essential for maintaining customers' involvement and interest. A frequent criticism from user and carer groups, who have assisted with the work of services, is that no change has taken place. Where customers see real change happening as a result of their input, the experience is likely to be more positive.

Questionnaires

Within services, questionnaires are frequently used, and frequently not returned. Most people using a learning disability service will have difficulty completing a questionnaire. Questionnaires are most effective when management and staff in organisations give encouragement and support to users to fill them in and when it is known that the organisation will give feedback.

Example

In 'They should treat you like an adult or a lady', North Manchester Community Health Council and North Manchester Self-advocacy Project attempted to gain the views of learning-disabled people on the health services which they received. Despite the use of pictures and accompanying guidance notes for helpers, there was an extremely poor response rate (only 25 out of 500 questionnaires were returned). In an honest and constructive report they suggest that:

1 Questionnaires should be well presented, easy to understand, and support for those surveyed should be available.
2 Any process of consultation will be lengthy and difficult, and should be fully funded.
3 A variety of media should be employed that do not require spoken or written language (for example audiotapes, video art, photographs).
4 If improvement is to be real, then awareness training in rights and other services is necessary.

Documentation

Documents often go hand-in-hand with services. Some staff use them; others groan at the thought of them. Often they are a statutory responsibility, or needed as evidence that policies and work have been carried out. However, to someone unable to read, they are useless, as well as worrying and embarrassing.

Graphics, symbols and cartoons

These can be useful in putting a message across, often focusing the whole group when used in meetings.

In collating information for this chapter the acid test for documents was to remove any written information and see how many people could guess the meaning. Some were extremely clear, particularly where larger cartoons or fuller graphics were used. Others portrayed a very small part of the whole meaning. While symbols and pictures can be helpful, it is important not to assume that their meaning will necessarily be clear without first being learned.

Example

An art and a music group in Manchester have recently begun to involve members in planning. As well as changing the format of the meetings, they have experimented with the use of graphics and photographs to increase understanding of the agenda, and to explain which person would be leading each part of the meeting.

Video and audiotapes

These are being increasingly used in Manchester, both to publicise initiatives and to record events. Videos have the disadvantage of being extremely time-consuming to create but are popular with many customers and have the advantage of being available to a wide audience once produced.

Example

In Manchester a member of staff has formed a video production group with customers and has used video creatively within the service to demonstrate projects, aid staff training, publicise events, record memories and apply for funding. Following a recent customer conference it was decided to channel energies into a video record of the event for each delegate rather than a visual booklet. (See also Chapter 14 on the use of video for service development.)

Focus groups and workshops

Without service staff to inhibit contributions, workshops and focus groups are popular and unthreatening to many customer groups. If advocates are used, they can be extended to include those unable to communicate in a group setting. However, in practice, advocates are few and far between, and groups often rely on the most verbal people to represent all the customers.

A range of creative media can be particularly useful within focus groups and workshops to develop wider thinking and provide a change of tempo: collage, drawing, role plays, videos, wall posters, photographs and pictures.

Examples

1 Across Manchester regular local consumer days are held as work-shops on a theme – for example, leisure opportunities, health, relationships.

2 Last year a series of six workshops were held in Manchester to find out customers' views on the Community Care Plan.

3 A focus group which met to discover how to improve the complaints procedure for customers enabled the Joint Service to develop plans and seek funding for an independent complaints advocate who would also work to increase understanding of consumer rights.

Interviews

While interviews are useful for gaining in-depth information and give opportunities to probe for further information, they rely heavily on verbal communication skills: they can be a difficult medium for all but the most vocal customers.

Example

Good Practice in Network Houses by Fieldworkers (Goodman, 1995) aimed to find out what users, carers and staff involved in fieldwork considered to contribute to good practice. Customers interviewed often knew the fieldworker and could give much information about what the fieldworker had done for them and whether they felt positively or negatively about the input, but none of them was able to give further opinions. Even with probing and rephrasing questions, it was difficult to obtain a more detailed response than 'Good' or 'Didn't like them' or 'They were nice'.

It does take longer to obtain good interview material from people who are not used to giving their views, who may think slowly, or who may have reasons for not trusting people in authority roles.

It can be less threatening to have customers themselves carrying out interviews.

Example

In *Outside But Not Inside Yet* (Manchester People First, 1995) two members of this advocacy organisation carried out research – much of it in the form of interviews – to find out the views of people moving from hospitals into the community.

Conferences

As with workshops, conferences gain a great deal of momentum from the energy created by bringing a group of like-minded people together and giving more weight to views expressed. They can often form the basis for support groups and the development of local consumer groups.

Examples

1 From a customer conference in one city, user forums were formed, regular feedback to management has been established and two customers are now members of the Social Services Committee.

2 In conjunction with People First, Manchester's Joint Service has recently held its first customer conference. This involved the use of an experienced workshop leader, independent of the service, who worked with customers and group facilitators over two days. Issues of concern were identified and recorded and, on the final afternoon, these were presented to a panel of senior managers from the purchasing and provider organisations. Three months later, a recall day was held during which a video of the event was shown and the panellists reported back on what they had achieved in responding to users' issues. The Joint Service plans to hold a customer conference annually.

Customer committees and local user groups

Within the framework of the all-Wales strategy, Clwyd included service users in local planning groups, and most services have users' committees with small budgets. Participation has been incorporated into training, along with workshops to find out views. Clwyd established a local policy framework whereby money for services was withheld if users were not represented.

Conclusion

All local authorities must involve customers in community care planning. Beyond this, the Manchester Joint Learning Disability Service is trying to develop a culture whereby its customers feel they possess both ownership of, and the ability to contribute to, the development of their service. It is an ongoing process which the Joint Service readily acknowledges to be at only an initial stage. By continuously learning more from its customers and shaping itself to encourage contributions, it will increasingly become the service its customers desire.

References and resources

Brandon, D., Brandon, A. and Brandon, T. (1995), *Advocacy: Power to People with Learning Disabilities*, Birmingham: Venture Press.
Burton, M. and Kagan, C.M. (1996), 'Rethinking empowerment: shared action against powerlessness' in I. Parker and R. Spears (eds), *Psychology and Society: Radical Theory and Practice*, London: Pluto Press.
Cocks, E. and Cockram, J. (1995), 'The participatory research paradigm and intellectual disability', *Mental Handicap Research/Journal of Applied Research in Intellectual Disabilities*, 8 (1), 25–37.
Croft, S. and Beresford, P. (1993), *Getting Involved: A Practical Manual*, Brighton: Open Services Project/Joseph Rowntree Foundation.
Dluhy, M. (1990), *Building Coalitions in the Human Services*, Newbury Park, California: Sage.
Feuerstein, M-T. (1986), *Partners in Evaluation: Evaluating Development and Community Programmes with Participants*, London: Macmillan.
Gomm, R. (1993), 'Issues of power in health and welfare' in J. Walmsley, J. Reynolds, P. Shakespeare and R. Woolfe (eds), *Health, Welfare and Practice: Reflecting on Roles and Relationships*, London: Sage.
Goodman, K. (1995), *Good Practice in Network Houses by Fieldworkers*, Manchester: Joint Learning Disability Service.
Illich, I., Zola, I.K., McKnight, J., Caplan, J. and Shanken, H. (1977), *Disabling Professions*, London: Marion Boyars.
Jack, R. (ed.) (1995), *Empowerment in Community Care*, London: Chapman and Hall.
Kagan, C. (1997) *Agencies and Advocacies*, Whalley, Lancashire: North West Training and Development Team.
Manchester People First (1995), *Outside But Not Inside Yet*, Manchester: People First.
Servian, R. (1996), *Theorising Empowerment: Individual Power and Community Care*, Bristol: The Policy Press.
Shearer, A. (1991), *Who Calls the Shots? Public Services and How they Serve the People who use them*, London: King's Fund.
Simon, K. (1996), *I'm Not Complaining But … Complaints Procedures in Social Services Departments*, London: Joseph Rowntree Foundation.
Whyte, W.F. (ed.) (1991), *Participatory Action Research*, Newbury Park: Sage.

17 Planning with people

Helen Sanderson

Introduction

The way in which a service approaches planning with people demonstrates how close it is to the values espoused in its mission statement. This chapter describes person-centred planning and how it requires a shift in thinking and practice for all staff and managers if people's lives are really to change. It describes what this can mean in practice and gives examples of how Manchester is working to change its practice and put disabled people firmly in the centre of the process.

From individual planning to person-centred planning

There are many different styles of individualised planning used in UK services, most of which originated from Individual Programme Planning (IPP) which was developed by Roger Blunden and colleagues in the early 1980s, drawing on the work of various North American workers (Blunden, 1980). Typically, individual planning has involved an annual meeting with a six-monthly review. The process usually begins with a meeting of the key people in the person's life, and the key worker presents information about the person and their strengths and needs. Goals – usually long-term and short-term – are discussed and agreed, and a review of these takes place six months later. Other approaches have been developed, which focus more on the person advocating for themselves and the quality of their life rather than what the service wants them to learn or change next. This process of shared action planning encourages people to take a greater role, make choices and set their own agenda with friends and family as well as service providers.

Whatever format is used, most people with learning difficulties have experienced planning where staff have assumed that they know what is best and set goals that focus on changing and 'fixing' the person. People have had little support or say in the planning process and were assigned to the most appropriate service depending on their disability or needs. Everybody received similar plans and similar options – usually with other people with learning difficulties. Little, if any, attention was given to other potential kinds of help from family, friends or neighbours. For some people this is changing; for many people, if planning happens at all, it is still a bureaucratic paper chase that results in little meaningful change in their lives.

Services that are trying to change are listening to what people with learning difficulties have to say about planning, investing in approaches to planning, known as 'person-centred planning', and focusing on involving people from the community.

Person-centred planning refers to a collection of techniques for getting to know the people involved, developing an understanding of what people want now and what they want their future to look like, and setting priorities for change. It also focuses on helping services to become more flexible and responsive and building bridges into the community. Person-centred planning is not about 'fixing' the person but about people coming together to solve problems, build and grasp opportunities, influence communities and change organisations. This takes place over a period of time and, although it usually begins with a process of getting to know the individual and an initial planning meeting, this is the start, not the end, of the process.

A variety of techniques has been described for use in person-centred planning, which include Personal Futures Planning, PATH, MAPs, and Essential Lifestyle Planning (ELP). Each involves getting to know the people involved and helping them to describe how they would like their life to be.

Services vary in the way in which they use person-centred planning. Some services have used it to replace their existing style of individual planning; others use it to amend or supplement their existing planning style; and others have used the approaches for people in certain situations. It must be emphasised that it involves a change in thinking about people and is not simply a new set of paperwork using colour and posters or a new planning technique. Some people even question whether services can embrace person-centred planning without it becoming another empty service ritual.

Moving towards person-centred planning requires some fundamental changes in how services get to know the person, involve that person in planning, in the way that the plan is created and, most importantly, in ensuring that change takes place as a result of this.

Practical guidance: what is the difference?

Getting to know the person

Moving from traditional planning to person-centred planning represents a significant shift in power – away from professionals being in charge of collecting and holding information and making decisions about the person's life. In person-centred planning the individual and the people who care about the person take the lead in deciding what is important to the person, which community opportunities should be taken or created and what the future could look like.

Professionals move from being the experts to being information providers adding to the overall picture of what is important to the person, what support they need and what they want for the future.

Table 17.1 compares the traditional, service-led approach with that of person-centred planning. It should be noted that the 'traditional approach' described here is something of a caricature, and the desirable approach is somewhat ideal in nature, but this has been done to identify clearly the direction in which it is important to develop these approaches.

Developing a vision and plan for the future

In existing, traditional ways of planning with people, the process often begins with professional assessments in which the person is described in terms of what they cannot do – in other words, their deficiencies. This tends to result in setting goals to try and 'fix' these deficiencies. One of the effects of this is that people are only given opportunities which staff feel that they are 'ready' for. In person-centred planning the focus is on dreams and visions of better lives for people, which are not limited by what the service has to offer but truly represent what is important and cherished by the person. However, to many people working in services this is seen as encouraging people to have unrealistic expectations and therefore setting people up for disappointment and failure. Certainly, stretching the imagination and the boundaries of what is possible will often result in frustration and disappointment, but it also may change lives beyond what was thought possible. This is not the

Table 17.1 Comparison of service-led and person-centred planning

Moving from	Moving towards
How do we get to know a person?	
Professional assessments are completed on the person. The person may never see the report of results of the assessment. His or her opinions are not sought or valued.	The person chooses someone to help them think about their life and record what is important to them. They spend time getting to know each other, finding out who they are, who is important to them, what they enjoy doing.
	More 'technical' knowledge from assessments would only be used within this context and done with the person and not on them.
How do we describe them?	
The person is described in terms of their label and what they cannot do (deficiency descriptions). This may include a 'strengths and needs' list completed by staff about the person.	Some people may record important things about their life in whatever way best suits them, using video, pictures, photographs or words. If the person does not use words to communicate, imaginative ways of representing what is important to them are used.
Information about the person is recorded for professionals only and is stored in files which are accessible only to professionals.	All descriptions of the person focus on what is important to them, and what they are able to do – their capacities and gifts.
	Where the person's problems and challenges need to be described, this is done in as constructive a way as possible.
	The person is encouraged to tell their own story, recorded in whatever way is most relevant to the person – video, photographs, audiotape or written.

simplistic process that it may sound. It requires open and honest discussion with the person and the other important people in the person's life.

The planning process is different when the person is truly at the centre, since whatever is needed to enable the person to participate as fully as possible is considered. This ranges from months of planning with the person to help them discover what is important and what their dreams are, to simply changes in hospitality to make people feel more at ease. It is not just the person him or herself who is encouraged to participate, but also family, friends and other people from the community whom the person has invited to become involved. These represent two of the most important challenges in person-centred planning: how can the person be supported to participate as much as possible, and how can we encourage and facilitate family, friends and non-service people to contribute? This means that more meetings have to take place at the weekend or in the evening and tests just how flexible services can be, or are willing to become, in order to take this process seriously.

Different styles of person-centred planning can be used. Some of the most well known are Essential Lifestyle Planning, PATH, MAPs and Personal Futures Planning.

Essential Lifestyle Planning

Essential Lifestyle Planning was developed by Michael Smull and Susan Burke-Harrison (1992) initially as a way of discovering what is important to people in their day-to-day lives. It is a way to learn:

- who and what is important to people in their everyday lives
- how to support people to have the lifestyle that they want
- how people can have what is important to them while staying reasonably healthy and safe
- how to change the service the person receives to reflect what is important to the person and how they want to live.

This information is recorded in a clear, simple but powerful way in the person's Essential Lifestyle Plan. The plan is developed by spending time with (and listening to) the person, and having conversations with other people who know and care about them.

PATH and MAPs

MAPs and PATH are graphic planning tools developed by Jack Pearpoint, Marsha Forest and John O'Brien (see Pearpoint *et al.*, 1993). They derive from an interest in building inclusive communities and provide a framework for translating idealistic visions into practical first steps which empower people and their allies for change.

Key steps in constructing a PATH involve answering the following questions:

- What is the dream?
- What are our goals?
- Where are we now?
- Who else do we need to involve?
- What do we need to do to stay strong and keep going?
- What are the first steps?

Personal Futures Planning

Personal Futures Planning was developed by Beth Mount and is a planning process that involves:

- getting to know the person and what their life is like now
- developing ideas about what they would like in the future
- taking actions to move towards this, which involve exploring possibilities within the community and looking at what needs to change within services.

The process is colourfully recorded in words and pictures using different 'maps' or 'tools'. Each part of the planning process is guided by what is important to the person and the five accomplishments, which help people to reflect on whether the decisions and choices being made will really contribute to a better quality of life or reinforce negative experiences (Mount and Zwernik, 1988).

Our Plan for Planning

Whatever style of planning is used, the principles of keeping the person at the centre are the same. People First groups in Liverpool and Manchester have contributed through the booklet *Our Plan for Planning* (People First, Liverpool and Manchester, 1996) which can be used as a first step in listening to how people want to be supported in planning meetings. It originated from consultation with the People First groups in Liverpool and Manchester as part of the Joseph Rowntree-funded People, Plans and Possibilities Project, and other People First and self-advocacy groups have had an opportunity to contribute to it. The booklet describes the support which people would like before, during and after their planning meeting – including what staff must *not* do. It describes ways of keeping the person in the centre of the process – one of the fundamental principles of person-centred planning. Table 17.2 compares the service-led approach to planning meetings with the person-centred approach.

Table 17.2   Comparison of the service-led and person-centred approach to planning meetings

Moving from	Moving towards
What is the purpose of the meeting?	
Meetings are organised to coordinate services and set goals for the person. They are also used to monitor the person's progress.	The meeting is organised to help the person identify what is important to them now, what they want for the future and what needs to happen to enable the person to achieve the life they want now and the future they desire.
How is planning organised?	
Every professional involved with the person is automatically invited to their planning meeting, which has been booked by the manager. The meeting takes place in the most convenient offices during normal working hours.	The person or their advocate decides who they want to be involved in helping them plan their future. These people are personally invited.
The person is just informed of the date, time and venue.	The person chooses the date and time of the meeting. They also decide on the venue – often their home, the community centre or a local room which can be hired. They get whatever help they need to do this.
What happens in planning meetings?	
The meeting is run by the manager or a professional involved with the person.	The meeting is facilitated either by the person themselves – with help if they need it – or a facilitator whom they have met before.
The planning group listens to professionals' reports.	When other people have something to say, it is presented in a way that the person understands.
The focus for setting goals is on improving skills and behaviour –	

Table 17.2   concluded

Moving from	Moving towards
'fixing the person'. Short- and long-term goals are set within the capacity of the service.	The person is supported by the group to clarify what is important to them, their dreams and what they would like their life to be like in the future. This may include experiences that they want to have, contributions that they want to make, new living arrangements or better relationships with people. The emphasis for the group is on listening to the person, to what they say and what their behaviour tells them. Goals are set which focus on helping the person achieve the life they want now and moving towards the future which they have described. This may involve actions for the person, their friends, family, neighbours or other people from the community.
What happens after the meetings? The staff who attend receive typed minutes. Little change takes place. The plan might be forgotten about until the next review.	The plan is reviewed every six months. The person is involved in recording the meeting. If the person does not read, they are given the plan/minutes in pictures, on tape or whatever way is most accessible to them. Their life changes as goals are achieved. The person and the group regularly review the plan as things change.

Building support and making change

Person-centred planning is a tool for helping people to start the ongoing work of helping people to achieve the life they want and to make their contribution to the community. Investing in the people who are going to help make that happen is essential if lives are really going to change.

The plan has to be seen as a living entity which grows and changes and does not wait, dormant, until shortly before the next prescribed review. It needs to be constantly revisited, through team meetings in which people can consider the progress that they are making as a group, by individuals considering with their managers, how their contribution to the plan is developing and, most importantly, by the person him or herself. As well as giving the opportunity to review the goals that were made at the meeting, the spirit of the dream and vision can inspire other actions that lead towards it.

Table 17.3 compares traditional service-led and person-centred support.

Table 17.3 Comparison of service-led and person-centred support

Moving from	Moving towards
Support group	
Inconsistent teams without any involvement of community people.	Person-centred teams where stability is enhanced by people other than those in staff roles.
How does the team relate to the person?	
Support staff are not encouraged to develop close relationships with the people they support, as this is seen as unprofessional/or becoming too involved. Staff are routinely moved every six months so that the people they support do not become 'dependent' on them.	Support staff are encouraged to develop good, lasting relationships with the people they support.
What happens to the plan?	
The plan is not referred to, and the actions tend to be left until a few weeks before the next meeting.	The plan is a 'living plan' and reviewed at team meetings, in job consultations/supervision to see how the goals are being met.

Table 17.3   concluded

Moving from	Moving towards
How are problems solved? Problems and difficulties are ignored until they reach a crisis, and then the plan or the person is blamed.	Problems are aired and resolved interactively with the person and the team.
How is the community involved? Very few ordinary community members are involved, and they are viewed with suspicion by the services. The team pay lip-service to welcoming advocacy but view other people's involvement as interference.	The team is constantly looking for ways of involving more community people in the person's life. Advocacy is taken seriously and welcomed, even when it results in criticisms of the service.
How does the team work together? Staff teams do not work well together, there is poor communica-tion and the focus is on bureau-cratic details rather than what is important to the person they are supporting	The person-centred team is united in its focus on how to improve the quality of life for the people they support. Attention is given to team-building and developing the team's individual strengths and interests.

Connecting people and communities

This involves a significant change in what services see as their most impor-tant role – to help people develop relationships and to participate in, and contribute to, their local community. This overarching aim, and what the person has described as being important to them in their plan, will provide the detailed goals. This requires that services refocus or completely change recruitment policies, training agendas and attitudes towards relationships between support staff and the people who receive a service. Table 17.4 illustrates this shift.

Table 17.4 Comparison of the service-led and person-centred approach to connecting people to their communities

Moving from	Moving towards

How important is developing relationships within the community?

Moving from	Moving towards
Support staff devote little time to helping people develop relationships and connections in the community.	Developing relationships is seen as a key area that people need and want help with. This is kept in mind with regard to all support given to the person.
Some support staff might even sometimes wonder whether the community is the best place for people to be, thinking that people are not made welcome and that there is nothing that can be done about that.	Staff receive training and development in helping them understand the importance of relationships and the community. This focuses on helping people look at how they developed their own network of friends and what their own community is like, and then considering how they can help the person become more involved in their community.
Staff are recruited and are assigned to work anywhere in the service, with no attempt to match them to service users' interests and needs.	Support staff recognise that helping people to feel at home and to be able to contribute to their local community requires commitment and imagination but is certainly possible and definitely worth the effort. They spend time discovering and thinking about the community and searching for ways of helping the person have a role in their local community. They invite people from that community to join them.
	Recruitment procedures recognise the importance of people living and working in their local community in order to support others to live and work in their local community.

Changing services

Person-centred planning can therefore be used to address both the short-term issues of improving the quality of the person's life now and the longer-term issues of achieving the person's dreams and aspirations. This begins the process of developing person-centred support and results in organisational and community change as the problems and challenges with which people have to deal are often the consequence of oppressive organisational practices or unwelcoming communities.

Table 17.5 Comparison of the traditional services concept and the person-centred services concept

Moving from	Moving towards
What do services value?	
They value standardisation, efficiency and cost-effectiveness above all else.	They value people being supported to have high-quality lives as well as local initiative, diversity and developing individual and flexible supports for people.
How are services seen?	
Services are seen as having all the answers to understanding and meeting the needs of people who require support	Services are seen as encouraging people from the community to work in partnership with the person and services to share problems and ideas for solutions. The preferred approach is to look to community resources to meet people's needs before involving specialist services.
How do services respond?	
Services obstruct people achieving the lifestyles they want by being bureaucratic and inflexible.

They provide the same services in the way in which they have always been provided. | The services listen to what people have to say and what they want from them and, where necessary, change in order to respond to this. |

Person-centred support can bring people together to create new community roles and relationships for people with disabilities, their friends and support workers. This can change and effectively redesign the service culture, mission and structure. Table 17.5 illustrates this.

Examples from Manchester

In Manchester, changes are being made to move closer to the practice that has been described. *Our Plan for Planning*, personal portfolios and profiles are being used with service users to help them plan their meetings; there are 'dream workshops' and meetings facilitated by People First to help people think about their future; and the whole service is moving gradually towards using Essential Lifestyle Planning.

Changing how people prepare for their planning meetings

Using Our Plan for Planning

This booklet has been widely distributed to support staff involved in helping people plan their own meetings. It is being used by both the individual and their key worker to prompt discussion about how people want to be supported, where and when they want their meeting and how information should be presented. There is a gradual move away from booking consecutive IPP meetings in the office meeting room and informing people that their meeting will be held in two weeks' time. Support staff also use a booklet developed by a speech and language therapist and a psychologist on how staff can help learning-disabled people who have difficulties in telling others what they want and how they feel. The speech and language therapists and People First are working on producing more information and training on the specific issues of involving people who do not use words to speak in their meetings.

Developing personal profiles

Some people have found it helpful to use a book to record and describe what is important to them and what they want to change with another person. A booklet has been designed and piloted with People First covering the following broad areas of relationships, places to go, important routines, dreams, roles and skills to learn and leaving room for people to record their lives through photos, pictures, collage or words.

Some people choose to describe their own life through an autobiography or personal portfolio. There are some similarities in the ways in which staff would help people to describe their life either for a portfolio or a profile, but the underlying purpose and structure of each one is very different. People develop personal portfolios to describe or record any aspect of their life for themselves, through video, pictures, objects or in any other way that the person chooses. Although this is not designed to be shared with other people at a meeting, some people do use part or all of their personal portfolio in their meetings to show others a specific area or aspect of their life. Manchester People First have produced a video describing how to make a portfolio and giving examples of seven people's experiences of doing this. Each network has a copy, and people are given the opportunity to borrow it and decide whether this is something they would like to do.

Dream get-togethers

Dream get-togethers are based on an idea of Helen Jones and Paul Taylor. They help people think about alternative lifestyles and develop aspirations for their own futures in a small group, using pictures, magazines and photos. They can take place over one or two days and involve people setting three specific, achievable goals at the end of the workshop. About three months later a follow-up day is held to which senior managers are invited to hear what people have achieved, the dreams which they still want to realise and their opinions on the workshop. The emphasis is on sharing ideas about possible futures with others, taking time to think about what options are available and then deciding on a few achievable goals to move towards their dreams. Several dream get-togethers have taken place in Manchester, and people have often used some of that information in their planning meeting.

Thinking about the future with People First

Manchester People First regularly spend time with other self-advocates either for a full or half-day to help people think about a specific area of their lives. One of these sessions – called 'I want to get out!' – involved thinking about places which people wanted to visit; another was about relationships and considered the following questions:

- What do we understand by the word 'relationships'? What other words do we use when we talk about relationships?
- What relationships do we choose?
- What relationships happen in our lives – for example, family and staff?

- How do we make relationships – what do we contribute and what do we get?
- What is different about 'paid' or staff relationships?
- What are the different levels of relationships?
- What kind of relationships do we want?
- What can we do to help us get these?

From this, people took ideas, and often pictures and descriptions of what they wanted, which they then used in their planning meeting.

Implementing Essential Lifestyle Planning

Person-centred planning can be used as one way of bringing about organisational and cultural change, but it needs to be part of an overall change process. The change process which is being used in Manchester involves a gradual shift to person-centred planning, a focus on developing person-centred teams, and a continual process of identifying what is stopping plans from being implemented and feeding this information to senior managers who can start to refocus the organisation. It draws on recent ideas from organisational theory and builds on a series of steps proposed by Kotter (1995). Although these are presented in a sequential way, some happen at the same time, and many have to be revisited more than once.

Establishing a sense of urgency

The results of an audit and asking people what they wanted indicated that change was identified as important.

An audit was carried out on all the goals that were set from people's individual plans. This showed that the majority of plans had no long-term goals and few goals related to developing relationships; most were focused on the areas of self-help and independence. Furthermore, the goals were written in very general terms, which made it very difficult to know whether they had been achieved or not. This audit was used to communicate to managers that change was required.

Focus groups were also established, in which people were asked what they thought of the existing way of planning and what they would like instead. A series of focus groups were held with service users, parents and carers, community team staff, direct support staff and managers. Representatives from each group then came together and the results were collated. They were surprisingly similar. People wanted a greater focus on advance preparation, to make information and minutes accessible to service users, less paperwork, shorter meetings, for people to be able to choose who came, changes to the venue and time of the meetings and, most importantly, what was promised in meetings to actually happen.

Forming a 'powerful guiding coalition'

The next step is to mobilise this sense of urgency into an alliance of people which can start to plan and make changes. In Manchester a group called the planning development group was formed. The development officer who had initiated the focus groups on planning presented the results to the Joint Service managers. They discussed forming a group to look at the implications of what people had said, and one of the Joint Service managers agreed to help form the group. Twelve people volunteered for this work. The manager and development officer chose people who represented different parts of the organisation, with an emphasis on direct support workers.

The group met and discussed what their role should be. They negotiated with the senior management group that this would not be an advisory group, but one which had the power to decide on the way forward for planning in consultation with users and staff, and that they would also be responsible for the monitoring and quality of the planning. They would be given time to meet each month to do this, would report regularly to the management group and would have priority for funding for training courses related to planning.

Keeping it on the agenda and building support

The planning group used existing meetings to discuss planning issues. Some of this backfired a little, as people thought that they needed to make quick changes in order to be seen to be doing something. Manchester has a standard which states that everyone should have a planning meeting once a year: this was audited in April and revealed that almost half of the service users had had their planning meeting in March! The manager's request that these meetings were more sensibly spread out through the year was interpreted as each network needing to hold at least two planning meetings per month. To ensure that this happened some managers asked their staff for planning meeting dates six months in advance, which obviously meant that service users had limited control over when their meeting was going to take place.

The planning group and Joint Service managers were able to enter into dialogue and debate with some of the originators and early adopters of person-centred planning approaches (for example, Smull, O'Brien, Segal and Lovett), and this helped in the development of understanding of planning issues, leadership and participative management.

With the help of an external facilitator, the planning group also ran a three-day planning event with four focal people from one network, who do not use words to speak. The follow-up day gave managers an opportunity to engage with people and their circumstances and see the difference that good person-centred planning and staff commitment made. By also inviting the chair of social services and senior officers of the health authority, the service demonstrated that it was developing a commitment to person-centred planning and generated interest in making sure that these developments continued.

Learning from our own experience and consulting with others

We considered different styles of planning and eventually decided that, for most purposes, Essential Lifestyle Planning was the most suitable system to aim for and we used it on ourselves, our friends and colleagues. Members of the shared planning development group each made their own Essential Lifestyle Plan and then planned with a work colleague, or friend or family member to learn more about the process. They attended PATH training, part of which involved completing their own PATH. One person attended a Personal Futures Planning course which, again, involved completing some of the maps from Futures Planning.

Five members of the group then used ELP with someone they supported and discussed with the group what they had learned from doing this, what the individuals themselves had thought about it and shared comments from friends and family members who were involved. The group also talked to specialists in the organisation – for example, specialists in work with behavioural challenges and speech and language therapists – to gain their opinions.

This process confirmed the group's confidence that ELP was the most suitable planning tool to be used across the service. They recognised that the service needed to learn, and gain a greater understanding, about the person individually and develop more continuity of support. The group also recommended that, once ELP was established within the service, they could move towards a 'tool box' approach, drawing on the other planning approaches as well as developing local techniques.

Having made these decisions, the group presented them to the rest of the Joint Service managers and arranged for these managers to spend a day with the group learning about ELP. During the day, each manager completed their own ELP.

Consultation also took place with the rest of the organisation and was instrumental in securing organisational ownership and backing for the development.

Creating a vision

Once the group is clear about the direction which it wants to take and has consulted on this with others, the next step is to develop it into a coherent vision.

The shared planning development group used the PATH planning process to develop their vision about the changes required and to plan exactly how they would achieve them. PATH also involves identifying who else needs to be involved or 'enrolled' to make this happen and setting milestone dates for the group to be able to monitor their progress.

Communicating the vision

This stage involves finding ways to communicate the vision to everyone throughout the organisation. The shared planning development group had identified all the stakeholders as part of the PATH process. They then identified how much each stakeholder needed to know about the process – for example, did they just need to know what ELP was or did they need to know how to facilitate a plan? Following this, they worked out how best to supply the person with the necessary information and who was to organise this. Part of this task involved getting copies of the PATH shared and discussed with each part of the organisation.

Empowering others to act on the vision

The shared planning development group established an ELP subgroup of people who had been involved in all of the initial ELP planning and pilot and who were developing their expertise in this area. Facilitator training was then organised for each assistant network manager and manager. Part of the facilitator training was to create 'your own ELP'. I took on the role of mentor for these facilitators, dealing with questions about the process. A series of meetings then followed with the ELP mentor and team broadly following the plan below. If individual team leaders were having difficulties, the mentor would try to arrange individual sessions to coach and support them.

Planning for and creating short-term wins

The group looked for ways in which they could build short-term wins in the early months of the PATH and how these experiences could be shared with the rest of the organisation.

Consolidating improvements and producing still more change

This is the 'long haul' stage of continuing to improve, encourage, empower and learn. It involves constantly evaluating progress and what needs to change. It also involves problem-solving and redesign, based on feedback.

The shared planning development group met regularly to review progress. Many situations arose which seemed to knock all the careful planning sideways – for example, industrial action and overtime bans.

Institutionalising new approaches

This stage involves looking for ways to embed the planning process in the new and changing culture.

Including ELP as part of induction programmes and service philosophy courses has moved this process forward, but it needs to have more far-reaching effects on policies, procedures and the use of resources.

The danger at this stage is that the organisation incorporates the new planning approach and reduces its radicalism, rather than undergoing change itself as a result of what is being learned from the planning process.

Continuing to learn and review

This stage continues the learning and review and seeks ways in which this can have a deeper and more lasting effect on the organisation's culture. The challenge is to continually evaluate how what is being learned from ELP can be used to inform and stimulate cultural change.

Monitoring and evaluating person-centred planning

One of the functions of any group that seeks to implement person-centred planning is to discover ways of:

- continually improving the planning which takes place
- discovering what organisational changes are required to gain more successful outcomes
- exploring ways in which people and community members can be more involved in the planning process
- reviewing the quality of the recording of the plans
- identifying training and support needs.

The shared planning development group looked for ways to obtain feedback about the way in which all individualised planning was happening, not just the first ELPs that were being developed. One of the assistant network managers pointed out that, in her job consultation with her manager, he rarely asked about planning, although there were structured evaluations of the condition of the house, finances and so on. Recognising that job consultations of this nature sent messages to the organisation about what was important and what was not and that it could seem as if planning was low on managers' agendas, the group designed a feedback form with the network manager.

At the job consultation, the manager and assistant manager went through the feedback form for a randomly selected individual in order to identify areas where planning could be improved. From this development, goals were set for both the assistant manager and the manager and reviewed at the next meeting.

Summaries of the findings are sent to the shared planning development group. The next steps for the group are to develop ways of evaluating the 'structure' of the plan, the process of planning and the outcomes from the plans.

Developing person-centred teams

Most person-centred plans are implemented by the team which supports the person, working with friends, neighbours and other people from the community who care about the person. Often the only people involved in making the plan a reality are service providers. The process of putting the plans into action is usually where the really hard work begins. The facilitator or assistant network manager is crucial to supporting and assisting the team to make the plan a 'living plan' which is constantly referred to and reflected on, changing as necessary without losing the central thrust. The Manchester Joint Service is beginning to look at the implications of building person-centred teams (see Sanderson, *et al.*, 1997).

Conclusion

Implementing person-centred planning involves rethinking how people are involved in their meeting, the planning styles used and strategies for keeping the plan 'alive'.

Building person-centred teams means using the same principles which are being encouraged in person-centred planning with staff. In organisational terms, this reflects what has been described as a 'learning organisation' which supports its staff to constantly reflect on their work, use their initiative and problem-solve together. It requires that an organisation devolves power down to the level where the action actually takes place, which would mean creating semi-autonomous teams who work with the manager to make decisions about the best use of the team's resources in order to support people to achieve their plans and achieve the life which they want.

Manchester is beginning to address these challenges as the organisation tries to change from a bureaucracy to a more participative and person-centred organisation.

Acknowledgements

I am grateful to Michael Smull and John O'Brien, for frameworks and advice on individual planning frameworks used in this chapter.

References and resources

Blunden, R. (1980), *Individual Plans for Mentally Handicapped People: A Draft-Proce-dural Guide*, Cardiff: Mental Handicap in Wales Applied Research Unit.

Brechin, A. and Swain, J. (1987), *Changing Relationships: Shared Action Planning with People with a Mental Handicap*, London: Harper and Row.

Burton, M., Kagan, C. and Clements, P. (1995), *Social Skills for People with Learning Disabilities. A Social Capability Approach*, Chapman and Hall, London 1995.

Burton, M. and Kagan, C.M. (1996), 'Rethinking empowerment: shared action against powerlessness' in I. Parker and R. Spears (eds), *Psychology and Society: Radical Theory and Practice*, London: Pluto Press.

Kotter, J. (1995), 'Leading change: why transformation efforts fail', *Harvard Business Review*, March–April.

Mount, B., and Zwernik, K. (1988), *It's Never Too Early, It's Never Too Late*, Minnesota: Paul Metropolitan Council.

O'Brien, J. and Lyle, C. (1986), *Framework for Accomplishment*, Decatur, Georgia: Responsive Systems Associates.

O'Brien, J. and Lovett, H. (1992), *Finding a Way to Everyday Lives*, Pennsylvania: Pennsylvania Office of Mental Retardation.

Pearpoint, J. (1990), *From Behind the Piano: The Building of Judith Snow's Unique Circle of Friends*, Toronto: Inclusion Press.

Pearpoint, J., Forest M. and O'Brien, J. (1993), *PATH: A Workbook for Planning Positive Possible Futures*, Toronto: Inclusion Press.

People First, Liverpool and Manchester (1996), *Our Plan for Planning*, Manchester: People First (Fourways House, 57 Hilton St, Manchester, M1 2EJ).

Sanderson, H., Kennedy, J., Ritchie, P. and Goodwin, G. (1997), *People Plans and Possibilities*, Edinburgh: Scottish Human Services.

Smull, M. W. and Burke-Harrison, S. B. (1992), *Supporting People with Severe Reputations in the Community*, Alexandria, Virginia: National Association of State Mental Retardation Program Directors.

Social Services Inspectorate (1996), *Planning for Life: Developing Community Services for People with Complex Multiple Disabilities. No. 2 Good Practice in Manchester*, London: Department of Health.

Wertheimer, A. (ed.) (1995), *Circles of Support: Building Inclusive Communities*, Bristol: Circles Network UK (35 Mangotsfield Rd, Mangotsfield, Bristol).

Appendix

Professional Supervision Framework

Mancunian Community Health (NHS) Trust
City of Manchester Social Services Department
Joint Learning Disability Service

Introduction and context

In the Joint Service all staff are accountable to a manager. For most professional staff (i.e. those in Community Learning Disability Teams) this is one of four team managers. Team managers come from various professional backgrounds and have a wide span of responsibility, so they cannot be expected to offer the support for and monitoring of professional practice. It is for this reason that all professionals will have a supervisor. Managers are expected to offer regular *job consultation* to their staff, while supervisors offer regular *professional supervision*.

Practice advisors and managers may delegate certain aspects of these functions to appropriately graded and experienced staff. In some cases it will make sense to delegate both functions to the same person (e.g. a senior therapist could supervise and manage key aspects of the work of a therapy assistant).

The rest of this paper identifies key aspects of good practice in professional supervision. A separate policy is available for job consultation.

Outcomes

Supervision should result in the following things:

For the staff member:
A sense of direction, with effort better focussed
Priority tasks set

Team Manager	Head of Profession (l.d.)	
(delegates function as appropriate)	(delegates function as appropriate)	
Appoints	Advises on appointment	
Recruits	Advises on recruitment	
Allocates work Defines parameters of work	Monitors appropriateness of work. Advises on appropriateness of work and its methods	*
Seeks understanding of approaches used and questions on lay, 'common sense' basis/ suggests alternatives	Challenges and supports specialised work content	*
Problem-solves re service coordination and provision	Problem-solves re work methods	*
Ensures adherence to employment and service requirements	Advises management on disciplinary matters that concern professional conduct	
Reviews effectiveness in relation to service goals	Reviews effectiveness in relation to best practice	*

* job consultation/supervision functions

Skill and knowledge increased about information, people, equipment, sources
Problems solved, or better defined
New ideas
Training needs identified
Increased confidence, with work problems and issues in appropriate perspective
Feel valued and affirmed
Further contact arranged
A summary record of the supervision session

For the supervisor:
  Knowledge of professional practice
  Practice evaluated and monitored
  Knowledge of the staff member
  Knowledge of the workload: scope, extent, content, pressures
  Knowledge re fulfilment of professional, and service standards
  Knowledge of development needs/training required
  Issues identified for management action
  Further contact arranged
  A summary record of the supervision session

For the service:
  Confidence that professional practice is monitored and supported effectively
  An organised approach to staff development, and career progression.

Content

Professional supervision should cover assessment, planning, treatment/direct provision/advice, recording, reporting and evaluation.

Information sources

The supervision process will be informed by direct observation, supervisee's verbal description of the work, documentation (in case files), and where available or appropriate, by feedback from colleagues and management.

Requirements

For the above to happen, the following requirements will need to be met:

1. There should be regular planned sessions without interruptions, with sufficient time, and a lack of undue pressure.
2. Supervision should not only be office based, but involve some observation of work practice, on the job coaching, and joint working, especially for more recently qualified and junior staff.

3. Contact between formal sessions (telephone, corridor, brief consultations) is desirable.

4. Formal sessions should lead to a legible written record, filed and available to both parties, and kept for a minimum of 24 months.

5. The content of supervision is confidential to the staff member and supervisor, except by mutual agreement (e.g. where an issue needs discussion with management), or very exceptionally, where other considerations require that others are made aware of particular information (e.g. issues of malpractice, danger to a third party, etc.).

6. There should be a review of conclusions at the end of a formal session.

7. The supervisor will be knowledgeable about the areas of professional practice covered (and will know and make clear any limits of her/his expertise). Since the supervisor is in an 'expert' role regarding the professional practice issues s/he will need reasonable access to relevant professional updating (books, journals, courses).

8. The supervisor needs the authority to change or even stop practice as well as to develop it.

9. The supervisor needs the interpersonal skill to establish rapport, and trust, and to be an effective listener and facilitator of the staff member in conversation.

10. The practice advisor (lead supervisor for each professional group in the service) requires some managerial skills of

delegation

understanding the service in its context

self organisation

11. The practice advisor will need accessibility to and from junior staff

12. The practice advisor will need regular access to management.
  i There will be at least annual joint appraisal meetings with supervisor and team manager.
  ii Practice advisors will have a regular meeting with each team manager (at least six-monthly).
  iii Practice advisors (and supervisors) will inform team managers of development and training needs.
  iv Practice advisors will give advice to senior management on career progression, grading, recruitment, and service development.

13. The practice advisor will require supervision or peer review

within profession

within speciality

and in some cases (for example where there is nobody available locally with the required knowledge and experience) this may need to be arranged with a senior professional from outside Manchester.

Monitoring

Practice advisors monitor supervisors within their profession.
Head of Development and Clinical Services monitors supervision by practice advisors (supervision practice rather than professional content)
Trust Heads of Profession outside learning disability services (where available) provide support on clinical and professional issues to practice advisors.

Minimum frequencies for supervision

(but in many cases will see staff more frequently, especially where the work is stressful, unfamiliar or particularly complex)

Staff experience/ grade	Examples	Minimum frequency
Senior	Nursing H and above Psychology B Speech and Language Therapy Grade 3 and above O.T. Head III	3 months
Experienced	Nursing F–G Psychology A (> 2 years post qual.) S & L Grade 2 (2 years post qual.) O.T./Physio. Senior 1 and 2 Care managers, level 3 social workers	1–2 months depending on experience
Recently qualified/ junior	Nursing D–E Psychology A (less than 2 years post qual.) S & L Grade 1 O.T./Physio, basic grade Care managers, level 2 social workers	monthly
Unqualified or part qualified staff	Nursing A–C Psychology Assistants Therapy Assistants Care managers (unqualified)	monthly

These frequencies are for guidance only and arrangements may vary to increase, or exceptionally to decrease these frequencies.

Printed and bound by CPI Group (UK) Ltd, Croydon, CR0 4YY

21/10/2024

01777086-0006